Detecting & Living with Breast Cancer

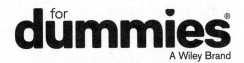

for
dummies®
A Wiley Brand

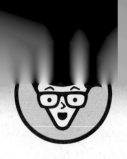

Detecting & Living with Breast Cancer

by Marshalee George, PhD, MSPH, MSN, AOCNP®, CRNP, and Kimlin Tam Ashing, PhD

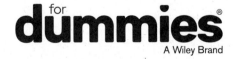

for dummies®
A Wiley Brand

Detecting & Living with Breast Cancer For Dummies®

Published by: **John Wiley & Sons, Inc.,** 111 River Street, Hoboken, NJ 07030-5774, www.wiley.com

Copyright © 2017 by John Wiley & Sons, Inc., Hoboken, New Jersey

Published simultaneously in Canada

For general information on our other products and services, please contact our Customer Care Department within the U.S. at 877-762-2974, outside the U.S. at 317-572-3993, or fax 317-572-4002. For technical support, please visit https://hub.wiley.com/community/support/dummies.

Wiley publishes in a variety of print and electronic formats and by print-on-demand. Some material included with standard print versions of this book may not be included in e-books or in print-on-demand. If this book refers to media such as a CD or DVD that is not included in the version you purchased, you may download this material at http://booksupport.wiley.com. For more information about Wiley products, visit www.wiley.com.

Library of Congress Control Number: 2017948467

ISBN 978-1-119-27224-3 (pbk); ISBN 978-1-119-27225-0 (ePub); ISBN 978-1-119-27226-7 (ePDF)

Manufactured in the United States of America

10   9   8   7   6   5   4   3   2   1

Contents at a Glance

Table of Contents

CHAPTER 18: **Making Healthy Lifestyle Changes**...................267

PART 5: THE PART OF TENS...285

CHAPTER 19: **Ten Inspiring Breast Cancer Survivors**.............287

Foreword

I am excited to write this foreword for *Detecting & Living with Breast Cancer For Dummies* by Drs. Marshalee George and Kimlin Tam Ashing. As a survivor, I believe that the comprehensive and easy-to-read information this book provides will help readers navigate each stage of their healthcare and personal journey from diagnosis to survivorship. In clear, concise language this book explains testing, procedures, and treatments that individuals experience. The authors understand the questions that concern patients at every stage and they deliver the answers in topical chapters.

For my fellow survivors, I encourage you to start by looking over the table of contents, which offers you an overview of the breadth and depth of coverage. This book tackles topics that we are sometimes hesitant to ask and even sometimes don't even know to ask. For example, chapters detailing surgical procedures, chemotherapy, and radiation demystify the experiences through patient-centered teaching. This book attends to social, family, sexuality, and psychological matters and is clearly intended for the whole person. It thoughtfully addresses medical communication and improving physical, social, and emotional well-being to "live our best life possible," as the authors put it. This empathetic, knowledge-based approach lives in each chapter and continues throughout the book.

Detecting & Living with Breast Cancer For Dummies is a powerful and compassionate resource.

—Nilaya Baccus-Hairston, JD, breast cancer survivor

Introduction

Welcome to *Detecting & Living with Breast Cancer For Dummies!* We wrote this book in association with the American Breast Cancer Foundation to help men and women live full and productive lives after a diagnosis of breast cancer.

The impact of a breast cancer diagnosis and its treatments can be challenging and sometimes even devastating for some breast cancer survivors. Some survivors report that they endure pain and physical and emotional problems, and that their family, sexuality, intimacy, and social and work lives suffer. But we are here to tell you that in doing our breast cancer survivorship clinics and community studies, we've met many hopeful, purposeful and resilient men and women.

Your authors Drs. George and Ashing, along with other colleagues, have examined quality care and coping among breast cancer survivors and caregivers throughout the breast cancer journey. A wealth of our clinical and professional experience has come from their work at their academic and NCI-designated Cancer Centers (Johns Hopkins Sidney Kimmel Comprehensive Cancer Center, Maryland, and City of Hope, Comprehensive Cancer Center, California). Our work is grounded in a multidisciplinary, whole-person approach integrating mental, physical, social, and spiritual aspects of breast cancer survivors' healing and recovery. We provide educational, quality care, research, and advocacy information and resources that strive to empower breast cancer patients and their loved ones. Given our interest and expertise in health disparities, this book attends to the unmet needs of ethnic minority, low-income, and underserved cancer survivors. As scientists-advocates, our efforts have contributed to breast cancer patient-centered research and best practices in their local communities, nationally as well as nationally and internationally.

The American Breast Cancer Foundation (ABCF) at www.abcf.org is a national 501(c)(3) charity providing educational resources, vital funding to aid in early detection, treatment, and survival of breast cancer for underserved and uninsured individuals, regardless of age or gender. ABCF addresses many issues and provides resources for many subjects that are addressed in this book.

As you strive for wholeness, remember that breast cancer is not your fault. With advances in early detection and treatments including personalized medicine (genetics, genomics, combination treatments, and immunotherapies), breast cancer is increasingly treatable and even curable. In this book, we offer you our cumulated wisdom on treatment decision making, self-care, hope, mindfulness, and healthy adaptive behaviors, so you can live your healthiest life possible.

About This Book

This book encapsulates both East and West Coast breast cancer experiences in the United States thanks to the clinical, research, and community experiences of both authors. The content of the book conducts the reader along their breast cancer journey, addressing questions they may have along the way and dispensing nuggets of wisdom to better their experience.

This book also draws from the personal stories of diverse breast cancer survivors from all walks of life, and pays attention to ethno-cultural diversity and inclusion in the delivery of care.

Each chapter not only focuses on part of the step-by-step process of getting diagnosed, deciding on treatment, and recovering from treatment, but also offers practical self-help strategies of dealing with sabotaging issues for healthy living.

Our aim is to take the reader into the breast cancer experience from diagnosis through treatment and survivorship. It is to be used as a reference, and you don't need to read the book from beginning to end, in order. Neither are you expected to remember everything.

This book aims to bring to the forefront issues that breast cancer survivors are concerned about beyond treatment. It's meant to be practical and address real-life issues related to breast cancer treatment through the eyes of survivors.

This book also has tips on managing psychosocial stressors, dealing with sexuality and fertility concerns, engaging in intimacy, making healthy lifestyle choices, and obtaining information on special communities.

Within this book, you may note that some web addresses break across two lines of text. If you're reading this book in print and want to visit one of these web pages, simply key in the web address exactly as it's noted in the text, pretending as though the line break doesn't exist. If you're reading this as an e-book, you've got it easy — just tap the web address to be taken directly to the web page.

Foolish Assumptions

We assume a few things about you, the reader, but not many. We assume you read at least at an eighth-grade level, have no medical background, and don't necessarily have any knowledge of breast cancer or its treatments. You may be newly diagnosed with breast cancer, receiving active treatment, recovering from treatment, or you may be several years out from treatment.

Perhaps you're a friend or family member who wants to support a loved one with breast cancer. Regardless of your situation, reading this book will help you discover all aspects of breast cancer treatment, including cutting edge treatments, innovations in breast reconstruction, how to live well after breast cancer, and much more.

Icons Used in This Book

The icons you see in the left-hand margins throughout the book are there to help you identify information that may be of particular interest in certain ways — or not.

TIP

This icon points out especially useful information or good practical advice for you regarding some aspect of breast cancer treatment and survivorship.

REMEMBER

This icon highlights information you would do well to tuck into your brain's file drawer for later use.

This icon lets you know there is something to especially watch out for or be cautious about.

WARNING

TECHNICAL STUFF

This icon points out peripheral information you can safely skip, that's not necessary to understanding the main point under discussion.

Beyond the Book

In addition to the material in the print or e-book you're reading right now, this product also comes with some access-anywhere goodies on the web. Check out the free Cheat Sheet by going to www.dummies.com and searching for *detecting and living with breast cancer*. You'll also find a downloadable, free survivorship care plan.

Where to Go from Here

Feel free to browse the table of contents to determine which chapter seems the most interesting to you. You don't have to read the chapters in order (although you certainly can, and they do build on each other in some ways). You can also check the index to jump straight to any particular topic you want to know more about.

If you're new to the subject and want to just begin somewhere, you can hardly go wrong by beginning with Chapter 1. If you're newly diagnosed with breast cancer, you might check out Chapter 14, which deals with psychosocial concerns after diagnosis.

However you use this book, we hope you find it useful as a guide to successfully navigate difficult situations. We also hope you find what many have found — that faced with the right attitude, surviving cancer can actually enhance your life, your relationships, and your sense of purpose in the world.

1

Knowing About Breast Cancer

Chapter **1**

Breast Cancer 101

The breasts are often viewed as one of the most feminine parts of a woman's body. After all, they're sexual organs as well as vital organs for feeding an infant. Touching the nipples stimulates the same areas of the brain as touching the genitals does. Stimulation of the nipple during breastfeeding increases the release of *prolactin*, a hormone made by the *pituitary gland* (a pea-sized organ in the center of the brain). The release of prolactin causes a woman's breasts to produce milk during and after pregnancy. It also stimulates the release of *oxytocin*, another hormone produced by the pituitary gland in the brain that causes the cells to eject or let down milk when the cells squeeze down on the milk ducts. This mechanism works with suckling of the infant to maximize milk discharge.

As we explore breast cancer and treatments in the upcoming chapters, we talk a lot about the different parts of the breast. Therefore, it's important right up front that you get familiar with the different parts of the breast and their functions. We break it down like pieces of a puzzle, and when the pieces are all put together, you will understand better what a healthy, normal breast should look like. Knowing the big picture will help you understand the changes that can occur in the breast, how those changes are diagnosed, how they are treated, and how to access the support you need from family, friends, and your healthcare providers throughout the process.

Knowing your breast, its parts, and functions, will help you

>> Spot changes or unusual symptoms.

>> Have better conversations with your healthcare providers.

>> Make more informed decisions.

>> Feel satisfied that you have received the best treatments.

Breast Cancer Basics

Let's start with the most fundamental biological unit: the cell. As you may (or may not) remember from biology class in school, the *cell* is the basic building block of the human body and is where life begins. A group of cells is called *tissue*. And a group of tissues is called an *organ*. The breast is considered an organ, like your kidney, spleen, and brain.

Finding your way around your breast

The breast extends from the collarbone to the underarm and across to the middle of the chest at the sternum. The breast is mostly made up of *adipose* tissue, which means it's a collection of fat cells. The size and number of fat cells in the breast are influenced by many hormones, genetics, growth factors, and lifestyle behaviors — and the female hormone *estrogen*.

The breast is divided into 12–20 sections called *lobes.* In these lobes are many small glands called *lobules,* which produce milk in nursing mothers. Milk *ducts* are small channels that collect the milk that is produced in the lobules and convey milk to the nipple. Throughout the adipose tissue of the breast is a network of ligaments, fibrous connective tissue, nerves, lymph vessels, lymph nodes, and blood vessels. Figure 1-1 shows the breast and some of its parts.

Here are a few more important parts of the breast:

>> **Areola:** Dark area around the nipple.

>> **Blood vessels:** Help carry blood throughout the tissue.

>> **Connective tissue:** Made up of muscles, fat, ligaments, and blood vessels. It provides support for the breast, gives shape to the breast, and separates or binds other tissues within the breasts.

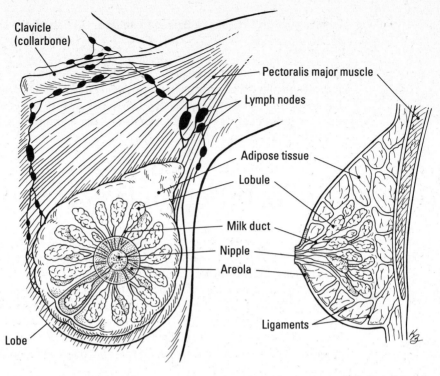

FIGURE 1-1: The illustrated breast.

Clavicle (collarbone)

Pectoralis major muscle

Lymph nodes

Adipose tissue

Lobule

Milk duct

Nipple

Areola

Ligaments

Lobe

Illustration by Kathryn Born

>> **Lymph nodes:** Small kidney bean shaped pieces of tissue that are connected by lymphatic vessels that are part of the immune system. They are located in various areas throughout the body and act as a filter for getting rid of abnormal cells from healthy tissue. The majority of the lymph nodes that filter the breast are in the underarm area (armpit).

>> **Lymph vessels:** Lymph vessels are a network of vessels running throughout the body. They are part of the immune system that transports disease-fighting cells and fluids.

>> **Nerves:** Provide sensation to the breast.

Knowing about breast cancer risk factors and indicators

It's not just women who are at risk for breast cancer — men are too. Everyone needs to know how to lower the risk of breast cancer, and that includes considerations for modifiable factors (things you can change) and nonmodifiable factors (things you can't change). Chapter 2 explores more about the known risk factors for breast cancer.

Even if you have one or more of the risk factors mentioned in Chapter 2, it doesn't mean you will get breast cancer. Many people have risk factors for breast cancer but never get it, and others who don't have risk factors do get breast cancer. The key is to know your risk factors for breast cancer and minimize them as much as possible to reduce your risk.

Distinguishing Different Breast Cancers

We've all heard the terms *tumor* and *cancer* thrown around. But is there a difference — and if so, what is it? Technically there is a difference, although many people use these terms interchangeably. A *benign* tumor or neoplasm is a mass that is generally harmless, as this is an overgrowth of normal tissue. An example would be a freckle or benign mole that grows on the skin, or the raised lumpy tissue that forms over a cut to create scar tissue. A *malignant* (cancerous) tumor is bad news, as this is an overgrowth of mutated tissue. A malignant tumor is also called a *cancer* (or malignant neoplasm). An example would be a mole that undergoes mutations to become a melanoma (a type of skin cancer).

When the term *cancer* is used, it refers to new malignant growths that have the ability to spread to surrounding tissues and organs. As cancer tissue grows it can begin to infiltrate and replace all the normal tissue which can prevent an organ, for example, from functioning. Cancer sucks the nutrients and blood supply from your body to itself through a process called *angiogenesis*. Angiogenesis is when new blood vessels are formed from your existing blood vessels that are necessary for cancer growth. The blood vessels carry oxygenated blood and nutrients to the cancer, causing the cancer to grow and eventually spread to other organs (metastasis), and this can lead to death if left untreated.

Understanding angiogenesis is a very important area of research. Some treatments for breast cancer, such as chemotherapy, focus on disrupting the blood supply to the cancer, causing cell death.

In medical terminology, the location of the cancer cells in the body determines what it's called. So, if the cancer is found in the breast, it's called *breast cancer*. There are different types of breast cancer that are defined by the part of the breast where the cancer is found. The different types of breast cancer are as follows:

>> **Ductal carcinoma (cancer of the milk ducts):** When cancer is found within the milk ducts of the breast, it is called *ductal carcinoma.* Ductal carcinoma is the most common type of breast cancer. It affects the lining of the milk ducts that carry breast milk from the lobules, where it's made, to the nipple. If the cancer is limited to the lining of the ducts it is called DCIS (ductal carcinoma in situ). When the cancer breaks out of the milk ducts and starts to infiltrate the rest of the breast, it is considered *invasive* or *infiltrating* ductal carcinoma. DCIS and invasive ductal carcinoma are illustrated in Figures 1-2 and 1-3.

FIGURE 1-2:
Ductal carcinoma in situ (DCIS).

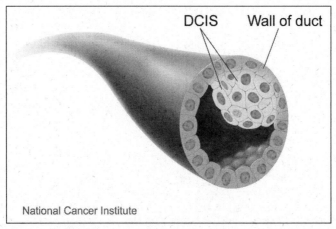

Illustration courtesy of the website of the National Cancer Institute (www.cancer.gov)

FIGURE 1-3:
Invasive ductal carcinoma.

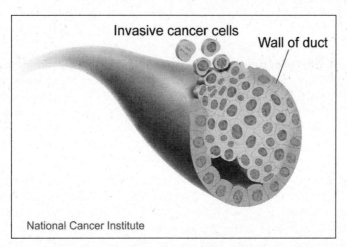

Illustration courtesy of the website of the National Cancer Institute (www.cancer.gov)

>> **Lobular carcinoma (cancer of the lobules):** When cancer is found within the lobules of the breast, where breast milk is produced, it is called *lobular carcinoma*. If the cancer is limited to a small area in the lobule it is called LCIS (lobular carcinoma in situ). When the cancer breaks out of the lobules, it is considered invasive or infiltrating lobular carcinoma.

>> **Inflammatory breast cancer:** This is a rare, aggressive form of breast cancer that often invades the lymphatic vessels and skin of the breast. It can be confused with an infection initially, as it will often cause an area of redness and swelling on the breast. See Figure 1-4.

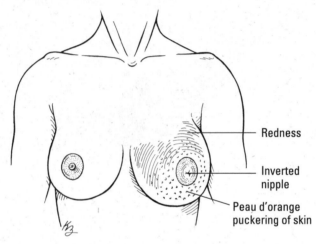

— Redness

— Inverted nipple

— Peau d'orange puckering of skin

FIGURE 1-4:
Inflammatory
breast cancer.

Illustration by Kathryn Born

>> **Phyllodes tumor (cystosarcoma — cancer of the connective tissues):** This is an even rarer type of breast cancer that doesn't usually spread to other areas of the body. There are two main types of phyllodes tumor: benign and malignant. No one knows what causes phyllodes tumors, but they appear to be more common in women with a history of fibroadenomas (benign breast lumps) and in women who are pre-menopausal between the ages of 35 to 50.

TIP

Cancer has the unfortunate tendency to not stay put, and when it travels, it brings destruction wherever it goes. When doctors find cancer in the breast, they immediately want to know whether the breast cancer has spread to the lymph nodes, and if so, how far it has spread. If the closest lymph node to the breast is found to have cancer cells, then additional lymph nodes are usually examined to determine if cancer cells are present.

WHY IS CANCER NAMED AFTER A CRAB?

The word *cancer* comes from the Latin word for crab. Why a crab? No one is sure. One theory is that it depicts the characteristic of the crab irregular shape with finger-like projections or claws that "don't let go." Crabs have eight legs on the back side of their body which helps to pull the crab to either the right or the left direction, making it impossible for them to walk in a straight line. This is similar to a cancer because its growth can't be controlled to be linear, horizontal, or vertical. Like a crab's legs, cancer seems to grow in any direction, and when the finger-like projections connect on a blood vessel or a tissue, they don't let go. They continue to invade more tissue. A crab will also keep moving, no matter what obstacle you may place in its way. This is also true for cancer. That's why it's often necessary to have multiple types of treatment, such as various chemotherapies, to kill the cancer. The treatments must aim to launch an attack on the cancer at every angle to weaken the cell and cause cancer death.

Lobular carcinoma in situ (LCIS), although it sounds like a cancer because it includes the term *carcinoma*, is *not* cancer. LCIS is a tumor that grows in the milk-producing lobules of the breast and remains inside the lobule — that is, it *does not spread* to other tissues. Unfortunately, having LCIS may increase your risk of developing invasive breast cancer in the future. In some people there may be a small area of malignant cancer hidden within an area of LCIS, which is why it has been recommended that LCIS be treated with surgical removal in certain people, depending on their other risk factors for breast cancer. Risk reduction treatment with endocrine therapy may be offered. See Chapter 11 for more information on endocrine therapy.

Detecting breast cancer

The diagnosis of breast cancer is multifaceted and includes changes that you may find on:

>> Breast self-exam

>> Clinical breast exam (done by your doctor or nurse)

>> Mammograms

>> Breast MRI

>> Breast ultrasound

See Chapter 4 for more information on the diagnosing process and testing for detecting breast cancer.

Biopsies and how they work

When a change in the breast is detected by breast imaging (such as by a mammogram, ultrasound, or breast MRI), a biopsy of the suspicious area will be recommended. Various types of biopsies are done according to the type of change seen in the breast (abnormal calcifications, breast mass, skin changes, and so on). Chapter 5 describes various types of breast biopsies and when they are used. A *biopsy* is a medical procedure that involves extracting and analyzing tiny samples of breast tissue for the presence or absence of cancerous cells.

TIP

You should discuss your biopsy results with your doctor or any other provider involved in your care (radiologist, gynecologist, or surgeon) even if you have received the written results and they indicate that you don't have breast cancer. Being informed of the status of your breast health will help you make the best decision for treatment with your doctor.

The pathologist and diagnosis

A *pathologist* is a physician who interprets and diagnoses the changes caused by disease in cells, tissues, and body fluids. The pathologist examines breast cells under the microscope to determine whether cancer is present or not.

Sometimes there are other changes in the breast tissue that might indicate that the tissue may develop cancer in the future, though cancer isn't present yet. Alternatively, a pathologist may see changes in the breast tissue that are completely benign and do not require any further action.

If cancer is detected, the pathologist must determine whether it is invasive or noninvasive. *Invasive* or *infiltrating* cancer is cancer that has spread from where it began in the breast to surrounding normal tissue. *Noninvasive* cancer has not spread outside the tissue in which it began. This is an important point, as it will often change the treatment plan.

Having an invasive cancer can dictate whether your doctor will recommend chemotherapy, radiation, or a specific type of surgery for you. Chapters 5 and 6 discuss types of biopsies and how to understand the findings of the pathologist for breast cancer staging. Breast cancer cells display various appearances under the microscope, and these appearances are used to distinguish the various types of breast cancer.

Grading and Staging of Breast Cancer

The grade and stage of breast cancers are determined by the pathologist based on how different the breast cancer cells are from normal breast cells and how quickly they grow.

Breast cancers are graded 1–3, with 1 being the most similar to normal, healthy cells, and 3 being the most different from your normal cells and most aggressive. Note that the *grade* of the tumor is a reflection of the pathology report and this is different than the *stage* of cancer.

Staging of breast cancer is determined from its size and location and whether the cancer has spread to other locations in the body. The size of a breast cancer can be measured in centimeters or millimeters. There are small and large cancers, and the size of the cancer doesn't always coincide with the aggressiveness of the cancer. Small cancers can be fast-growing, and large cancers can be slow-growing. Small cancers can be invasive, and large cancers can be noninvasive.

Sometimes cancer can occur in multiple areas of the breast (called *multi-centric*) or it can be in one location in the breast (*multifocal*). Chapter 6 talks more about the stages of breast cancer.

Planning Your Treatment

After the breast has been biopsied and breast cells have been examined by a pathologist, a *diagnosis* is usually made that lets you know what type of tumor is in your breast. Is it benign or is it malignant (cancer)? Knowing what you have is, of course, necessary for you to obtain the right treatment at the right time and at the right place.

Looking at your treatment options

If you have a diagnosis of breast cancer, it will require care from your cancer team who are specialized in different areas of medicine to treat you. This is also called a *multidisciplinary* team. Here are the usual members of a cancer care team:

>> **Breast surgeon (surgical oncologist):** A doctor who performs biopsies and other surgical procedures in breast cancer patients.

>> **Medical oncologist:** A doctor who specializes in diagnosing and treating cancer using chemotherapy, hormonal therapy, biological therapy, and

targeted therapy. A medical oncologist also gives supportive care and may coordinate treatment given by other specialists.

>> **Oncology nurse:** A registered nurse who specializes in treating and caring for people who have cancer.

>> **Oncology nurse practitioner or nurse practitioner (NP):** A registered nurse who has additional education and training in how to diagnose and treat disease and who is licensed at the state level and certified by national nursing organizations. In cancer care, a nurse practitioner may manage the primary care of patients and their families, based on their specialized training.

>> **Pathologist:** A doctor who identifies diseases by studying cells and tissues under a microscope.

>> **Physician assistant:** A health professional who is licensed to do certain medical procedures under the guidance of a doctor. A physician assistant may take medical histories, conduct physical exams, take blood and urine samples, care for wounds, give injections, and manage the care of patients and their families, based on their specialized training.

>> **Radiation oncologist:** A doctor who specializes in using radiation to treat cancer.

>> **Radiologist:** A doctor who specializes in creating and interpreting pictures of areas inside the body using X-rays, sound waves, or other types of energy. Many radiologists perform biopsies; if they do, they are called interventional radiologists.

>> **Social worker:** A professional trained to talk with people and their families about emotional or physical needs, and to find them support services.

Considering breast surgery

Breast surgery is a procedure used to remove the cancer from the breast. There are various types of breast surgery, including lumpectomy, mastectomy, axillary node dissection, sentinel lymph node dissection, and more. These are discussed in detail in Chapter 8. A surgeon will recommend the right surgery based on the size of the cancer, the size of the breast, whether the cancer has spread to lymph nodes under the arm, and patient preference.

TIP

The decision for which type of breast surgery should take place is ultimately the patient's — in other words, it's your decision. But you must be informed of all the breast surgical options available to you with consideration for the risk and benefits before making a decision.

Treating breast cancer with radiation

Radiation is a treatment option often used in conjunction with a lumpectomy as standard of treatment. The radiation beam is directed to the area where the cancer is located (while sparing surrounding healthy tissue) to kill any microscopic cancer cells that may have remained at the surgical site. See Chapter 9 for more information on types of radiation, how they are used, and when radiation is recommended.

Treating breast cancer with chemotherapy

Chemotherapy is a treatment option that uses various types of medicines that go to work on the various stages of the cell cycle. Chemotherapy medicines are given in combination, so when the cancer cell starts to divide and goes through the various stages of the cell cycle, the specific medicines activate at that cycle for maximum cell death. See Chapter 10 for more details on chemotherapy.

Treating breast cancer with endocrine (hormonal), biological, and other cutting-edge therapies

Endocrine therapy is also called *hormonal* therapy. Endocrine therapy is used to decrease estrogen in the breast tissue in the following situations:

» To reduce the size of the breast cancer (neo-adjuvant therapy or treatment before surgery).

» To reduce the risk of cancer coming back.

» To reduce the risk of cancer developing in individuals who are at high risk for breast cancer. (See Chapter 2 for more information on individuals at risk for breast cancer.)

Biological treatments are types of treatment that target specific receptors on tumors. These are protein molecules or biomarkers that can case the cancer to grow. Biological treatment is part of *personalized medicine* because it is given to individuals based on the actual characteristics of their breast cancer cells.

See Chapter 11 for more information on endocrine and biological therapy.

Treating advanced breast cancer

More and more individuals are living five, ten, or more years after being diagnosed with advanced breast cancer, thanks to innovative medicine and researchers and scientists looking for better and effective ways to manage advanced breast cancer as a chronic disease. Treatment for advanced breast cancer may include ongoing chemotherapy, endocrine therapy, biological therapy (that includes targeted therapy, monoclonal antibodies, and immunotherapy), and new innovative medicine in the form of clinical trials. Vaccine therapy has been very promising and may play a major role in the future in precision medicine (using your own genetic information to treat your cancer). Chapters 12, 13, and 14 talk more about treating advanced breast cancer and cutting-edge treatments.

Chapter **2**

Risk Factors for Breast Cancer

et us start by debunking the myth that you only get breast cancer if it is in your family. Despite this popular belief, approximately 87 percent of women diagnosed with breast cancer have no family history of breast or ovarian cancer. In other words, if you don't have a family history of breast cancer, you are in that 87 percent category of women who just might be diagnosed with breast cancer in a lifetime. So, every woman is at risk, but the cause of the risk may vary.

With that out of the way, this section covers some of the characteristics that do affect who is more at risk for breast cancer.

Advanced Age

The number one risk factor of any type of cancer is age. The older people get, the more incidences of cancer will be found. In the United States, we are becoming a more aged society, with the baby boomers getting older and living longer. With advanced age, there is ample time for breast cells to be altered or mutate due to internal genetic errors. Just like an aging car, some of the parts of a cell are subject to wear and tear over time and as a result function less efficiently. Additional risk factors like environmental exposures and poor lifestyle behaviors can increase your risk, as discussed later in this chapter. Table 2-1 shows how often women get diagnosed with breast cancer (incidence rate) and the age of diagnosis.

TABLE 2-1   **Estimated New U.S. Female Breast Cancer Cases by Age and Death**

Age	Noninvasive Cases	Invasive cases	Deaths*
<40	1,650	10,500	1,010
40–49	12,310	35,850	3,690
50–59	16,970	54,060	7,600
60–69	15,850	59,990	9,090
70–79	9,650	42,480	8,040
80+	3,860	28,960	10,860
All ages	60,290	231,840	40,290

*Rounded to the nearest 10. Data from American Cancer Society, Surveillance Research, 2015

Gender

It's surely not surprising that women are far more at risk than men for developing breast cancer. Males and females are both born with breast tissue, but the naturally elevated testosterone levels in males prevents the growth of mature breast tissue. This leaves males with a small amount of underdeveloped breast tissue. Male breast cancer makes up about 1 percent off all breast cancer. Chapter 17 talks more about men and breast cancer.

REMEMBER

About 12 percent of women in the general population have a lifetime risk for developing breast cancer. That's around one in eight women. For men, the lifetime risk for breast cancer is much lower: around one in a thousand.

Besides females having higher levels of estrogen than men, other risk factors can increase breast cancer in both male and females. Male risk factors for breast cancer are similar to risk factors in females, and although estrogen increases breast cancer risk for women, when women have certain diseases or are exposed to environmental toxins, their risk for breast cancer is much higher. Factors that might increase estrogen levels in males can also increase their risk of developing breast cancer.

The following are shared risk factors for breast cancer in both men and women:

>> **Being older:** The average age when men get breast cancer is between 68 and 71 years. For women, it's 50 to 69 years.

>> **Inherited gene mutations:** The mutation defect in BRCA 1 or BRCA 2 can increase the lifetime risk of getting breast cancer to 6 in 100. Both men and women may carry the gene. We talk more about genetics later in this chapter.

>> **Liver disease:** Cirrhosis of the liver can cause male hormones to be reduced, which can ultimately increase female hormones. In females, liver disease causes estrogen levels to surge to significantly higher levels.

>> **Alcohol:** Heavy drinking can affect the liver, increasing the risk of breast cancer.

>> **Radiation exposure:** If a man or woman has received radiation to the chest wall for cancer (for example, for lymphoma) they may develop breast cancer later in life.

>> **Obesity:** Fat cells convert androgens to estrogens in men when they are overweight, especially in the abdomen. In women, the fat cells may convert to estrogen, placing the body in estrogen overload.

Here are risk factors for men only:

>> **Testicular disease or surgery:** If his testicle is diseased or has been removed, then the man is more at risk for developing breast cancer.

>> **Occupation:** Working in industries that require men to work in a heated or hot environment, such as steel mills, or in jobs with increased exposure to gasoline fumes, can affect testicles, thus increasing risk for breast cancer.

>> **Klinefelter syndrome:** This occurs if a boy is born with more than one copy of the X chromosome, causing him to have more female hormones.

Race and Ethnicity

Even though White women (Caucasian and of European heritage) have a slightly higher risk for developing breast cancer over age 45, Black women — those of African American, African, and Afro-Caribbean descent — are more likely to die from the disease. The reasons for this are very controversial. Research in past years has shown that Black women have a higher incidence of *triple negative* breast cancers (see Chapter 5), though in clinical practice, cancer providers may observe differently. We provide care to equal numbers of both races of women with triple negative disease; the only common denominator is that the women are younger (under the age of 50). The verdict is still out on the true incidence according to ethnicity with triple negative disease. Several ongoing studies at the National Cancer Institute and NCI-designated cancer centers should help inform us in the near future.

Black women are also more likely to have higher grades and stages of breast cancer — in other words, they tend to have breast cancer that has spread to the lymph nodes under the arm and elsewhere, in comparison to White women. Research has shown that the driving factors in the higher incidence of breast cancer in Black women under 45 years are genetic mutation, family history, environment, lifestyle, socioeconomic status, cultural factors, and barriers to care. Lack of access to mammograms, delay in follow-up of abnormal mammogram results, denial of breast symptoms, competing priorities (single mother, other illnesses, and so on), lack of trust in the medical system, and financial limitations are all concerns for higher rates of breast cancer in Black women under 45 years.

Asian, Hispanic, and Native American women have a very low risk of developing breast cancer and dying from the disease.

For men, breast cancer is more common in White men than in Black men and least common in Asian men.

Information on breast cancer risk factors for Hispanic women is limited, even though they are the fastest-growing minority in the U.S. Hispanic women are quite often diagnosed with advanced breast cancer in comparison to non-Hispanic white women. The most perceived risk factor for breast cancer in Hispanics is less use of mammography screening in comparison to Black and White women.

Hispanics can have a lower risk of breast cancer if they have the gene ESR1. Research has shown that Hispanics are a heterogeneous population because they often have American Indian and European ancestry. When postmenopausal Hispanic women were tested in a U.S./Mexican breast cancer health disparities study, many Hispanic women were found to have the gene ESR1, which is typically found in Native Americans and which lowers the risk for breast cancer.

Overall, the risk of breast cancer typically increases in women who migrate to countries with high breast cancer incidence rates (such as the United States) from other countries with low incidence rates.

Early Menstruation and Late Menopause

Women who began their menstrual period before age 12 have a slightly higher risk for developing breast cancer than women who started after age 12. Similarly, those who go through menopause after age 55 years have a higher risk for developing breast cancer. This is believed to be because the more years a woman is exposed to sex hormones, the more at risk she is for breast cancer. The bodies of women who start menstruation early and finish late have been exposed to natural estrogen, progesterone, and testosterone for a longer period.

For the same reasons, *nulliparous* women (women who have never given birth to a child) and women who give birth to their first child after 35 years old also have increased risk of breast cancer.

Use of Birth Control Pills

If you take oral birth control pills, you may have a slightly higher risk of developing breast cancer in comparison to women who have not used them. However, when you stop taking or have discontinued birth control pills for at least ten years, your risk for breast cancer decreases and eventually returns to baseline (no increased risk).

TIP

You must take the time to discuss your risk for breast cancer with your GYN (gynecologist) when deciding to take birth control pills. Depo-Provera is a birth control shot that can be given as an alternative to birth control pills. The Depo-Provera shot is given every three months. It can increase your risk of breast cancer, but that risk is gone when you stop taking the shots for at least five years.

Genetic Risk: BRCA1 and BRCA2 Genes

Knowing your family history is very important to help determine your risk for breast cancer. You should do some research to figure out which family members had what type of cancer, on which side of the family (paternal or maternal), and at what age they were diagnosed with cancer.

If your first-degree relative (mother, father, sister, or brother) had breast cancer or ovarian cancer (females), your risk of having breast cancer is at least five times more than the general population without a family history of breast cancer. Your risk for breast cancer can be even higher than than that if your first-degree relative was diagnosed under age 50.

Tracing your family tree (genogram) is always helpful in providing a visual picture of family members who have had a history of cancer. It can also help providers to identify where the cancer clusters are in the family and which cancers you may be at risk for.

BRCA1 and BRCA2 (BReast CAncer susceptibility) genes are found in both men and women. When functioning normally, these genes produce special types of tumor suppressor proteins to repair damaged DNA in our cells. However, sometimes these BRCA genes are altered or mutated, and the proteins don't function normally. Sometimes damaged DNA is not repaired correctly, and then the cells are more likely to further develop with genetic changes that can lead to the development of cancer.

The BRCA mutation is detected by a genetic test, blood test, or from saliva, one of which is usually recommended if you have a family history of breast and ovarian cancer. The BRCA-mutated gene can be passed from your mother or father to you or siblings. If one of your parents has the gene, you have a 50 percent chance of inheriting the mutation. The two main types of BRCA genes, called BRCA1 and BRCA2, are both associated with an increased risk of female breast and ovarian cancers, and their presence accounts for 10 percent of all breast cancers and 15 percent of all ovarian cancers. When you have the BRCA1 or BRCA2 mutation, you are at risk for developing breast and ovarian cancer at a much younger age than other women who do not have the mutation.

It is important to note that not every person with breast cancer needs genetic testing. Individuals are tested for BRCA1 and BRCA2 mutation based on their genetic risk that assesses personal and family history factors, such as the following:

>> Breast cancer diagnosed before age 50

>> Cancer in both breasts in the same woman

>> Multiple breast cancers in the same woman

>> Both breast and ovarian cancers in either the same woman or the same family

>> Two or more primary types of BRCA1- or BRCA2-related cancers in a single family member

>> Male breast cancer

>> Ashkenazi Jewish ethnicity

TIP

If your family history is suggestive of a possible BRCA1 or BRCA2 mutation, the best thing to do is first test the family member with the known breast cancer. If that person is found to have a BRCA mutation, then other family members should consider genetic counseling to understand their potential risk for breast and ovarian cancer.

If you were adopted or otherwise don't know your family history and are diagnosed with breast cancer or ovarian cancer under age 50, it will be beneficial for you to consider genetic testing for BRCA1 and BRCA2. This will help you determine your risk for having a recurrent breast cancer or ovarian cancer, as well as your risk of passing it to the next generation (if you have or plan to have children).

WARNING

If you have either the BRCA1 or BRCA2 mutation, there are recommended measures you can take to reduce your risk of breast and ovarian cancer according to the National Comprehensive Cancer Network (NCCN) guidelines, as follows:

» Screening for breast cancer:

- Observe your breast for changes, starting at age 18

- Have a clinical breast exam performed by your doctor or nurse every 6 to 12 months starting at age 25

- Have a screening breast MRI annually, starting at age 25 or 30

- Consider a 3D tomosynthesis mammogram

- Screen after age 75 according to individual choice

» Reducing breast cancer risk:

- Consider removing the breasts (mastectomy)

- Consider risk-reduction medications (endocrine therapy: tamoxifen, anastrozole, letrozole, and so on)

» Reducing ovarian cancer risk:

- Remove the ovaries and fallopian tubes at the end of childbearing age

- Postpone removal of ovaries and fallopian tubes until mid-forties, especially in individuals who have completed risk-reduction mastectomies on both breasts

- Annually screen for ovarian cancer with the use of blood test CA-125, and transvaginal ultrasound if recommended by your doctor, starting at age 30

If you choose not to follow the risk reduction recommendations, you will be 7 times more likely to get breast cancer and 30 times more likely to get ovarian cancer before age 70 than women who do not carry the gene.

Note that there may be other genetic mutations that are inherited (passed on) to family members that lead to breast cancer. This is rare, but there are families with multiple members who have breast cancer that do not have the BRCA1 or BRCA2 mutation. It may be that scientists have not yet discovered the gene involved. At this time, the BRCA1 and BRCA2 genes are the ones that have been studied the most and are the most common cause of inherited breast cancer.

Poor Nutrition

When we are getting sufficient calories for energy and sufficient nutrients to support body function and growth, we can say we have good nutrition. Maintaining good nutrition and normal body function is a kind of balancing act. Our food must include a variety of fruits and vegetables, grains, fiber, protein with small amounts of fats, and lots of water to maintain good nutrition. Your body makes great efforts to fight off many diseases on its own, but it must have the right resources on its side to be able to do that. Poor nutrition reduces mental function and productivity as well as diminishes your body's immunity against diseases such as cancers.

REMEMBER

The best health outcomes occur when good nutrition is combined with regular physical activity. One hundred and fifty minutes of moderate exercise per week can lower your risk of breast cancer. No vigorous or intense exercises are needed to reduce your risk — if you walk for 30 minutes daily, your risk for breast cancer can reduce by 3 percent.

We all know that exercise can keep you at your ideal weight. When you're overweight, you have more fat cells or *adipose* tissue, which can release high levels of estrogen into your body. In general, obesity increases women's risk for any hormone-related cancer such as breast and endometrial cancer. Men who are overweight have an increased risk of prostate cancer.

Exercise is great for lowering insulin levels, hormones, and proteins (known as growth factors). Growth factors must be present for any cancer to grow.

Exercise reduces stress by releasing the brain's feel-good neurotransmitters, the endorphins. More endorphins reduce the urges to smoke and drink alcohol, which reduces your overall risk of breast cancer. Researchers have found that high levels of stress can damage your immune system, which can increase your risk of developing cancer.

Fats

Breast cancer cases are rarer in countries where the native diet is plant-based or vegetarian and very low in fat. Studies have shown that if girls eat a high-fat diet during puberty, they are at increased risk for developing breast cancer — even though they may not be overweight.

WARNING

But let's be frank about the sequence of events that in many cases leads to breast cancer. A high-fat diet means increased calories, and increased calories cause weight gain, which leads to obesity and increased levels of estrogen — which increase your risk of breast cancer. The next section talks more about obesity.

The relationship between diet and risk of cancer can be difficult to understand because diets consist of a variety of foods and nutrients, many of which can affect your cancer risk. Chapter 19 has more information on nutrition.

Red meat and processed meats

A diet rich in red and processed meats can increase your risk of cancer, whereas a diet rich in fruits, vegetables, and grains lowers your risk of cancer. Several researchers have found that the red pigment (called *haem*) in red and processed meat causes harm to the cells in the stomach and the bowels. Haem has its own toxicity but also promotes the formation and release of carcinogenic N-nitroso compounds (NOCs). It can also cause the production of toxins from bacteria in the stomach, which may lead to increased risk of various types of cancer such as breast, stomach, and colorectal cancer. Nitrates and nitrites are chemicals often used in processed meats and to preserve meat. When these chemicals are ingested and absorbed in the stomach and bowels, they can be converted into NOCs. This is likely why researchers have found a higher risk of cancer with processed meats in comparison to red meat. Research is ongoing into linkages between NOCs and other cancers such as breast cancer.

Who doesn't love to grill and barbecue? Unfortunately, researchers have also found cooking meat at very high temperatures produces cancer-causing chemicals called polycyclic amines (PCAs) and heterocyclic amines (HCAs).

TIP

Boiling or braising (frying lightly) and then stewing meats slowly in a covered container are great alternatives and may reduce the risk of cancer. Also, note that white meats (such as poultry, rabbit, and veal) contain very little or no haem, and the risk for cancer is low from eating white meat.

Obesity

Being overweight or obese can increase your risk of breast cancer when you are menopausal by 30 percent. Having extra fat in your body after menopause increases the production of estrogen and growth factors because the ovaries are no longer producing hormones and the fat tissue becomes the source of estrogen for the body. When the ovaries were producing hormones, they produced a regulated amount that the body needs for its function. But when the fat tissue produces estrogen, the amount is not regulated, and the body can be "flooded" with high levels of estrogen — which can lead to breast cancer.

In short, the increased risk of postmenopausal breast cancer is thought to be due to increased levels of estrogen in obese women. Because obese women have more fat tissue, their estrogen levels are higher, potentially leading to more rapid growth of estrogen-responsive breast tumors.

An increase in waist size before menopause may also increase your risk of breast cancer after menopause — separate from the obesity issue. Often, the body mass index, or BMI, is used to determine healthy weight. BMI is a useful tool for finding out if you are at a healthy weight for your height.

REMEMBER

BMI is only a guide and is not accurate for some groups of people, such as pregnant women, children, or people of African descent (due to increased bone marrow density).

Calculating BMI is done by a BMI calculator that factors in the weight and height of an individual. BMI calculators are widely available online. When you calculate your BMI, the following are the usual determinations of weight status:

>> BMI under 18.5 is underweight.

>> 18.5–25 is healthy weight.

>> 25–30 is overweight.

>> 30–35 is obese.

>> Over 35 is morbidly obese.

Again, BMI is merely a guide. Various ethnic groups have different BMI characteristics. Different individual lifestyles can increase bone density and lean muscle, thus causing someone to weigh heavier than the predicted weight on a BMI chart. This is why some women of African descent may weigh more than Caucasian women yet wear the same size clothing.

TIP

A simple, less accurate tool (widely used in the U.K.) that can help determine healthy weight is to simply measure your waistline. Use a tape measure to measure an inch above your belly button. A woman's waist should be less than 31.5 inches, and a man's waist should be less than 37 inches.

Smoking

Smoking can cause many types of cancer — primarily lung, throat, esophagus, bladder, and kidney — but it also has a small risk for breast cancer. Smoking cigarettes exposes the body to chemicals such as benzene, polonium-210, nitrosamines, and benzo(a)pyrene, which are known to cause DNA damage to tumor suppressor proteins that protect cells from developing cancer. Many cigarettes include the chemical chromium, which produces toxins like benzo(a)pyrene, which sticks to DNA like crazy glue and increases the amount of damage to proteins and cells. Other chemicals found in cigarettes include arsenic and nickel, which block the cells' natural process of repairing damaged DNA. It is for this reason that damaged cells are more likely to become cancerous.

Smokers' lungs are compromised, and they are less likely to tolerate exposures to toxic chemicals than nonsmokers with healthy lungs. The chemicals found in cigarettes make it difficult for smokers to remove toxins naturally because their immune system is weakened.

Alcohol Use

Consuming alcohol can also increase your risk of cancer. Whether you drink beer, wine, or spirits, no type of alcohol is better or worse than the other. Drinking alcohol and smoking together also increases your risk significantly for cancer. There is no "safe" amount of alcohol that you can drink if you want to prevent cancer, even though the American Cancer Society has stated that when you consume less alcohol, you reduce your risk of cancer. It's true that research has shown that one glass of red wine per day can help prevent heart disease — but not cancer. Short of stopping drinking altogether, the best action cancer-wise is to drink alcohol with caution and in moderation.

WARNING

The bottom line is that if you are accustomed to drinking a large glass of wine or a premium beer daily, you are increasing your risk of throat, mouth, esophageal, breast, and bowel cancers.

When alcohol enters the body, it is converted into acetaldehyde, a toxic chemical that is known to damage DNA and stop the tumor suppressor genes from repairing the damage DNA in cells. Acetaldehyde can also increase the growth of liver cells, thus increasing the likelihood of cells regenerating with changes or mutations that can lead to cancer. Our body also gets ethanol (another form of alcohol) from the foods that we eat, which is mainly broken down by the liver. Bacteria that live in the mouth and stomach can convert ethanol into acetaldehyde.

Alcohol also increases the levels of estrogen in the body. High levels of estrogen in the body can serve as signals for the cells to divide more rapidly, and that can increase the risk of breast cancer.

Prior Treatment and Chemical Exposures

If you have received mantle radiation or radiation therapy to the chest wall for Hodgkin's disease or any other disease, you may be at risk for developing breast cancer in the future. This history of prior radiation increases the risk of breast cancer because the breast is located in the field or area of the body where radiation was given.

Many individuals who have breast cancer with no family history have *sporadic* breast cancer. Research evidence has shown that the causes of sporadic cancers are largely attributed to environmental exposures such as silica and industrial fumes.

Exposure to DES (diethylstilbestrol)

If you were given DES (diethylstilbestrol) to prevent a miscarriage between 1940 and 1971, you have an increased chance of developing breast cancer. Additionally, if you were exposed to DES while your mother was pregnant with you, then you have a slightly increased risk for developing breast cancer after age 40.

Hormones: Estrogen and progesterone use

We have several types of hormones in our bodies, but the most important hormones for female organs are estrogen, progesterone, and testosterone — all produced by our ovaries. The various changes in hormonal levels in the body is what helps to regulate the menstrual cycle and all associated premenstrual syndrome (PMS) symptoms. When the levels of these natural hormones are higher than what they should be to regulate normal body functions, the risk for cancer increases.

Hormone-replacement therapy (HRT) is a treatment that is offered to women after menopause to treat menopausal symptoms such as hot flashes and mood swings. HRT replaces the natural hormones that the ovaries are no longer producing after menopause and can consist of a synthetic form of estrogen, called estradiol, or progesterone (called Norgestimate or norethindrone or drospirenone), which may be given as a single agent or in combination.

TIP

There is strong evidence that the use of HRT can increase the risk of developing breast, uterine, and ovarian cancer. However, it is important to consult your GYN to determine how taking HRT can benefit and affect your risk for cancer.

Environmental factors

There has been a public outcry in the U.S. and U.K. concerning manmade chemicals in food, household products, and the environment. Some of these concerns have focused on chemicals called *hormone mimics* and *endocrine-disrupting chemicals* (EDCs) such as phthalates or triclosan. EDCs are found everywhere. They are in pesticides, plastics, solvents, affected food, water, and vehicle exhaust fumes. People are exposed to EDCs by eating and drinking, using certain cosmetics and skincare products, and breathing in air. EDCs are found to disrupt the normal function of hormones in the body, which can lead to diseases that include cancer.

The air on any given day can consist of different substances depending on the types of pollution at your location, the weather, and the time of the year. Air pollution can come in the form of manmade fumes from smoking, vehicle exhaust, burning fuels from industries, as well as from natural sources such as radon gas, a natural radioactive gas. Radon is found in the air at a low level outdoors, but it can sometimes build up to high concentrations indoors.

Although chemical and air pollution are known to cause DNA damage to cells in our body, there is still insufficient evidence to link pollutants to specific cancers. We look forward to updates from ongoing research in this area of concern.

Even though this chapter has discussed some of the grim facts about what increases your risk of breast cancer, just know the following:

>> One out of eight women get diagnosed with breast cancer

>> Breast cancer is being detected earlier

>> Better breast cancer treatments are helping to cure and increase survival rates

Chapters 4 and 5 talk more about detecting breast cancer, and the chapters in Part 3 discuss the various ways of treating breast cancer in detail.

Chapter **3**

Indicators of Breast Cancer

Knowing your breast is the key to identifying changes that may be a sign of breast cancer. Sometimes fear can keep us hostage and prevent enjoyment of our health and life, and the fear of breast cancer is no exception to the rule. Understanding the signs and symptoms of breast cancer is essential for early detection of breast cancer and other noncancerous breast disease.

There has been great innovation and advancement in the treatment of breast cancer over the last few decades. The treatment for early stage breast cancer is usually less harsh, and most people go on to have normal and long lives with this treatment. That's why finding any changes in your breast and talking with your healthcare provider at the earliest point are very important.

REMEMBER

If you want to be a master of identifying breast changes, you have to examine your breast on a regular basis. Only you will know when something new has developed in or on your breast. Changes in the breast can occur from puberty throughout older adulthood, so you must ensure that every change noted on the breast is followed up with your doctor. Do not fall into denial and put off an examination if you feel something new in your breast. Go have it examined by a doctor. Early detection is important.

There are five main symptoms to look out for that could be concerning for breast cancer. Note that changes that only occur on one breast are more concerning for cancer, whereas changes to both breasts at the same time are less concerning:

>> Change in the size, shape, or feel of the breast

>> Skin changes

>> New lump in the breast or under armpit

>> Changes in the position of the nipple

>> Pain in your breast

REMEMBER

Know your breasts, so you can detect breast changes early.

Monitoring Changes in Breast Size and Shape

The size and shape of your breast are unique to you. Breast growth is mostly influenced by the release of estrogen and other hormones in your body, along with your genes (DNA) that you inherit from your parents. Your breast shape and how it looks are influenced by many factors:

>> Your age

>> History of childbearing

>> Breastfeeding

>> History of breast infections

When a female has passed puberty and the breasts are fully developed, that doesn't mean that the size of the breast will always be the same throughout her lifetime. For example, changes in your breast can occur after breastfeeding. The sucking effect from the baby on your nipples and the weight of the breast from full milk ducts can cause the ligaments that hold the breast against the chest wall to stretch. The skin can lose elasticity, connective tissue may be lost, and the breast shape may change to more of a tear-drop shape.

TIP

A good supportive bra is essential to reducing the effects of gravity on our breasts. *Yo-yo* dieting (in which you lose weight for a while and then gain it back, lose again, gain again, and so on) can also cause your breasts to droop because of the rapid weight loss and weight gain that stretches the skin. If this happens to you, doing exercises such as the dumbbell bench press (lie face-up with your arms straight, a dumbbell in each hand) and push-ups can help a little because having defined chest wall muscles may help give the illusion of perky breasts (though the actual breast tissue won't change as there are no muscles in the breast).

Breast increasing in size

Sometimes as an adult woman, you feel that your breasts are growing in size. This is often due to weight gain. Breasts, after all, are made up of mostly fat cells, and fat cells are also located in various other parts of the body. When you gain weight, the fat cells increase in numbers all over your body and form *adipose tissue*, which stores energy in the form of fat and cushions and insulates the body. Adipose tissue is also in the breast.

Pregnancy can make your breast larger because of the enlarged milk ducts to support breastfeeding. Birth control pills can also enlarge the size of your breast due to the increased sensitivity the breast has to hormonal changes (estrogen and progesterone) during your menstrual cycle.

TIP

When your breasts become larger, don't try to fit in the bra that you had last year. It's time to get measured and fitted for a new bra. This will ensure that the breasts are well supported and you are comfortable. If only *one* breast changes in size or shape, it's important to see your healthcare provider as soon as possible. If *both* breasts change in size and shape at the same time, it is most likely not due to breast cancer.

Breast decreasing in size

Your breasts tend to shrink when you lose weight, when you stop taking birth control pills, and when you become post menopausal — that is, when your ovaries no longer produce estrogen.

WARNING

If you have shrinking breasts along with hair loss, increased facial hair, or acne (on face, chest, and back), it may be because of high levels of testosterone and didehydroepiandrosterone (DHEA), which is the most abundant steroid hormone in the body. DHEA is produced by the adrenal glands, gonads, and the brain to enhance the function of androgen and estrogen in your body. It is important that you speak to your doctor if you're having these symptoms. You may need to be tested for polycystic ovary syndrome (PCOS).

There have been small studies that looked at the effect of caffeine on breast size. But there is no medical consensus on the effect of caffeine (in specific amounts) on breast size. There is no proven link between caffeine consumption and breast cancer at this time.

Watching for Skin Changes

Normally the skin on the breasts is a similar color to the skin on the rest of the body, thought it may be lighter due to less sun exposure. The nipple and areola (the dark area around the nipple) are usually a darker color with some bumps and textures. Just like the rest of the skin, there may be freckles or moles on the breasts. Some people also have stretch marks on their breasts due to changes in size over time.

Rash

You may develop a rash on the breast and be concerned because you wonder if it is inflammatory breast cancer. The best thing to do when you develop a rash is to talk to your doctor about it. Rashes can often be due to sweating and rubbing of skin surfaces together (also called *chafing*), and this most commonly occurs on the underside of the breast.

Another common cause of skin rash is exposure to new fabrics or products. Let your doctor know if you have a new bra, new skin cream, or new laundry detergent. If you can't determine the cause of a rash, the doctor may prescribe a topical steroid ointment or antifungal or antibacterial cream. The majority of skin rashes are not due to breast cancer.

WARNING

If the rash persists after treatment by your doctor, then you need to have further evaluation by a skin or breast specialist to determine if it is another breast condition or breast cancer.

Paget's disease

Paget's disease may appear as a rash around the nipple, especially on the areola. It's often mistaken for eczema or dermatitis. In addition to the rash, Paget's disease may involve the following:

>> Itching, tingling sensation or redness of the nipple and/or the areola

>> Inverted or flattened nipple

>> Nipple discharge that may be bloody or yellowish in color

>> Dry, scaly, flaking, crusty, or thickened skin around the areola

Many times the symptoms of Paget's disease are mistaken for those of another skin condition. It's often misdiagnosed, leading to delays in treatment. Many patients with Paget's disease often have breast cancer deeper in the breast, usually DCIS or invasive ductal carcinoma, which is why it's important to see your healthcare provider about persistent rashes on the breast. Treatment for Paget's disease is similar to breast cancer and may include breast-conserving surgery (lumpectomy) and radiation therapy. Explore Chapters 8 and 9 for more information on breast surgery and radiation therapy.

REMEMBER

If a rash on the breast is related to breast cancer, it will never go away — it either stays the same or gets worse after topical medication treatment.

Skin thickening

In *skin thickening* of the breast, the skin may appear to be swollen or filled with fluid and may have a ridging pattern resembling the texture of an orange peel (sometimes called *peau d'orange,* meaning "orange-peel skin").

Although skin thickening is one of the signs of inflammatory breast cancer, for it to indicate cancer there are typically other signs that most often occur together to confirm the diagnosis:

>> Redness over the breast

>> Breast feeling warm

>> Breast becoming harder

WARNING

If you experience *any* skin thickening on the breast, contact your doctor to have those symptoms evaluated.

Cellulitis

The breast may become red if there is a skin infection (called *cellulitis*). Cellulitis can often occur after radiation therapy or breast reduction surgery because these treatments can cause inflammation in the skin. Any inflammation of the skin can increase the risk of secondary infection.

When the cellulitis is due to infection, it's caused by bacteria that have gotten into the skin through a broken barrier, such as a wound. The infection can spread quickly, producing inflammation in the layers (dermis and subcutaneous tissue) of the skin. As the white blood cells in the immune system fight the infection, increased blood flow is seen at the site in the form of redness.

You may experience pain, tenderness, and swelling at the breast site and may develop a swollen lump or enlarged lymph node under the arm. The lymph nodes tend to get large closest to the area where there is an infection. This is a sign that the body's defense system (the immune system) is activated.

If you experience these symptoms, you must notify your doctor so you can be treated with an appropriate antibiotic.

Mastitis

Mastitis is similar to cellulitis in that the breast may become painful, red, and warm to the touch. However, mastitis is due to an infection deep in the skin, in the mammary gland (the milk-producing gland in the breast). It is due to bacteria getting into the breast via the nipple or a break in the skin. Mastitis most often occurs along with cellulitis of the breast skin. Other symptoms that may occur with mastitis include headache, fatigue, fever, and chills.

Breast abscess

A *breast abscess* is a hollow space in the breast that is filled with pus. This is due to infected milk ducts or an infection from the skin, which is caused by bacteria that get into the skin from the nipple or a break in the skin. *Staphylococcus aureus* is the most common bacteria found in breast abscess. Both cellulitis and mastitis (see the preceding two sections), if left untreated, can develop into a breast abscess.

Other factors that predispose a person to developing an abscess are diabetes and smoking. Smoking causes vasoconstriction and limits oxygen to the breast tissue for healing, thereby causing a delay in healing and risk of prolonged infection.

Most breast infections are treated with an antibiotic to kill *Staphylococcus aureus*, as this microbe is the most common cause. If the infection is due to a different bacteria, then the antibiotics may not help and the infection can get worse. If that happens and the infection gets worse a few days after starting antibiotics, your antibiotics need to be changed. Once an infection has an abscess, the abscess will need to be drained with a needle or surgically, in addition to taking antibiotics.

Breast infections are most common in women who are breastfeeding or who have recently stopped breastfeeding. Breast infection is caused by a break in the skin or the nipple that bacteria can get into. That means that a cut or scratch in the skin as well as a bite on the nipple can be the access point for the bacteria to get into the breast.

Breast infections do *not* cause or increase your risk of breast cancer.

Checking Out Lumps and Bumps

Sometimes we have to be like Sherlock Holmes when it comes to investigating changes in our breast beneath the skin. Lumps, bumps, and mass-like structures can develop in the breasts. Breast cysts and dense breasts are frequent findings on mammograms and breast ultrasounds. This section discusses their differences.

Breast masses and fibroadenomas

Often when a woman feels a lump or a mass in the breast, the instinct is to panic. However, 70 percent of masses or lumps found in the breast are benign — noncancerous. These benign masses are often harmless and may not require any treatment if they don't cause pain.

A fibroadenoma is a common benign mass found in the breast. It may cause the following:

>> Increase in breast size

>> Breast pain (*mastalgia*)

>> Lumpiness or hardness in the breast, especially before menstrual period

Fibroadenomas are well-rounded, smooth, and movable solid lumps that often develop outside the milk ducts and are most common in young women. They can develop in both breasts, and each breast can have multiple fibroadenomas. Fibroadenomas can get larger or disappear on their own. Fibroadenomas often grow larger during pregnancy.

No one knows what causes fibroadenomas. Because fibroadenomas increase in size and become painful especially during menstrual cycles, researchers have linked them to an abnormal hormonal response (specifically estrogen) in the breast tissue.

Breast cysts

Your breasts may feel lumpy all the time or only throughout your menstrual cycle. Lumpy breasts may be caused from dense breast (see upcoming section), hormonal changes, or PMS that increases the formation of benign (non-cancerous) *cysts* — fluid-filled sacs in the breast. Breast cysts inside the breast may feel like round balls with smooth edges. Some have described breasts cyst as feeling like grapes or small water balloons.

You can have cysts in one or both breasts, and there may be uneven numbers of cysts in each breast. Breast cysts may become tender or more painful just before and throughout your menstrual period or they may be painful all the time.

Treatment for a painful breast cyst may include *aspiration* — removal of fluid with a fine needle — or non-steroidal anti-inflammatory therapy (for example, ibuprofen, Aleve, and similar medicines).

REMEMBER

Talk to your doctor if you have a breast lump, so you can receive the best treatment. Tell your doctor when you first felt the lump, whether it has increased in size, whether it is painful, and what increases the pain. This information will help your doctor determine the next steps or testing that is right for you.

Dense breasts

REMEMBER

Many women think that a *dense breast* is when their breast feels firm and compacted, but that's not the case. Dense breast is *not* determined by how your breast feels or the breast size; it's *only* determined from the results of a mammogram. Chapter 4 talks more about mammograms.

On a mammogram, dense breasts are seen to have more fibrous and glandular tissue. Both cancer and dense breast tissue produce a white appearance on an X-ray.

TIP

Women with dense breasts should ask their doctor whether they need a 3D digital tomosynthesis (called a *3D tomo,* for short) for additional screening or for their next annual breast cancer screening, instead of a regular 2D mammogram. Chapter 4 talks more about 3D tomo screening mammograms. It is currently recommended that women with extremely dense breasts have a breast MRI and/or breast ultrasound for further evaluation during breast cancer screening.

Dealing with Breast Aches and Pains

Breast aches and pains are cause by compression of the nerve endings in the breast. Basically, neurotransmitters in the nerves send messages to the brain that the breast hurts. Anything that causes the nerves to be compressed can cause breast pain, including a breast mass, breast cyst, fluid/inflammation (which can be caused by infection or trauma), and scarring.

WARNING

A poorly fitted bra can also cause breast pain because it compresses areas of the breast, and fluid may be trapped in certain locations that compresses the nerve endings. Not wearing a good supportive bra while running or engaging in high-impact exercises can cause trauma to the chest wall and breast. Chest wall tenderness can last for several weeks because the muscle is strained. If you experience any of these symptoms, talk to your doctor to be treated.

Iron deficiency can also cause breast pain, due to iron's function of regulating thyroid hormones. There have been studies showing that 6 mg of an iodine supplement can reduce breast pain and boost thyroid function. If you have breast pain and think it is caused by iodine deficiency, you should discuss with your doctor to determine whether iodine supplements are best for you.

Nipple Changes

You should also watch for changes in your nipples. This section outlines some things to watch for.

Nipple inversion

Sometimes women may naturally have inverted nipples — in which the nipple does not protrude. That is their normal. But for some women, one of the nipples may become inverted or retracted when their normal is having "outies." If this happens, it is important to see your doctor, as it may be a sign of breast cancer.

TIP

But before you run off to the doctor, make sure your nipple wasn't temporarily inverted because of chest compression from a sports bra. If that was the cause, the nipple will pucker out eventually and was not related to breast cancer.

Milky nipple discharge

And when we hear the words *nipple discharge,* we usually think of pregnancy and breastfeeding. But it's normal for a milky discharge to continue for up to two years after stopping breastfeeding. There are other times that nipple discharge may occur outside of breastfeeding and pregnancy.

Nipple discharge can occur during or after sexual stimulation that includes foreplay or sucking on the breasts. It also can be caused by medication use. Breast milk is enabled by a hormone called prolactin, produced by the pituitary gland in the brain. Prolactin is regulated by dopamine, and when certain medications interfere with the level of dopamine in the brain, that can lead to elevated prolactin levels. Such medications include the following:

» Phenothiazines

» Selective serotonin reuptake inhibitors (SSRI), more commonly known as antidepressants

» Metoclopramide

» Risperidone

» Estrogens

» Verapamil

An underactive thyroid can cause also prolactin level to increase and cause nipple discharge. Kidney disease and stress can also elevate your prolactin levels. At the extreme is a noncancerous adenoma (tumor) called *prolactinoma* in the pituitary gland that increases the production of prolactin. Milky discharge is not commonly seen in breast cancer, but if you do start having discharge you should see your doctor to determine the cause.

Bloody nipple discharge

Very often women think that nipple discharge means they have cancer, but most nipple discharge is from noncancerous causes.

Bloody nipple discharge is often caused by a small noncancerous (benign) tumor called *intraductal papilloma* (IP) that is formed in the milk duct of the breast. IP is made up of fibrous tissue, glands, and blood vessels and is common in women between the ages of 35 and 55. IP can occur in one breast or both breasts at the same time and does *not* mean you have breast cancer. However, sometimes IP can contain abnormal or atypical cells, and these cells may increase your risk of breast cancer.

IP is usually painless, but because of the risk that it contains abnormal or cancer cells, the treatment recommendation is to have it surgically removed. Once the tumor is removed, it can be examined in more detail and determined if there are any areas of cancer within it. Most often there is no cancer associated with IP, but it is important to make sure. If you are diagnosed with IP, talk to your doctor to discuss the treatment best for you.

TIP

If you've had nipple discharge and wondered why the doctor kept asking you about the medications you were taking and ordered several blood tests, now you know that it was to determine whether your

>> Prolactin level was normal.

>> Thyroid function was normal.

>> Kidneys were functioning well.

>> Medications could be causing increased prolactin.

In addition, your doctor may order a mammogram, breast ultrasound, and/or breast biopsy (see Chapter 4 for more on these) to help confirm the diagnosis of IP.

WARNING

Nipple discharge is more suspicious for breast cancer when it only involves one nipple and when it occurs along with skin changes. You must seek medical care if you develop nipple discharge along with skin changes.

OTHER SKIN CHANGES

Color changes in the breast tend to occur often during pregnancy, when the nipple and areola often get larger and darker. The nipples and areola can also get darker as you age.

The breast may also change color with advanced breast cancers that may show the skin redder, darker, or dimpled. This occurs because cancer cells can block lymph vessels, which causes swelling.

2

Diagnosing Breast Cancer

Find out how to do a breast self-exam, what breast cancer screening guidelines mean, and how diagnosis works.

Get up to speed on breast biopsies and how they work.

Check out the stages and grading of breast cancer and what they mean.

Chapter **4**

Physical Awareness and Detecting Breast Cancer

Chapter 3 discusses the importance of knowing your breast and identifying changes that may occur with it. In fact, you should be aware of all body changes or symptoms. Periodically take a careful look at your body and especially at your breasts. Be proud of your body. We are all different, which means that the shapes and sizes of our breasts and body are unique to us.

Detecting breast cancer begins with you. And at a certain age you should undergo breast cancer screening, which usually involves the completion of a mammogram to determine whether there are any problems with the breast and whether additional diagnostic testing should be performed.

TIP

Exactly at what age breast cancer screening should begin is the topic of many deliberations among public health organizations and advocacy groups, but 40 is a good ballpark age to start asking your doctor whether you need a mammogram.

TIP

The better you know your breasts, the easier it is to identify when a change occurs, and the faster you can contact your doctor for an evaluation. It is important for you to know your family history, practice regular breast self-exams, and have timely mammograms as you get older, so that if there is a change in your breast, it will be detected early.

Believe it or not, there is no "right" or "wrong" way to check your breasts for changes. This section covers a few methods. You can check your breasts when you are in the shower, lying in bed, applying lotion, or getting dressed. Choose the method that is most comfortable for you. Once you choose a method, it's important to use the same one each time so you become familiar with how your breasts feel in a certain position. This will help you notice any changes over time.

REMEMBER

Everyone's breasts look and feel different. Some have lumpy breasts, large breasts, one breast larger than the other, or very small breasts (A cup size or they can fit a training bra). The areola may be large or small in size, and the nipple can naturally be flat, pulled in (inverted), or very raised — and they may have been that way since birth or became like that during breast development in puberty.

Self-breast exams are controversial, due to USPSTF, Susan G. Komen, and the American Cancer Society no longer recommending self-breast exams in their guidelines. Still, approximately 43 percent of breast cancers are detected by a mass felt in the breast during self-breast exam. In clinical practice, we have seen men and women who present with a breast mass that they felt, and when the mass was evaluated, breast cancer was confirmed. If these men and women were not performing self-breast exams, they would not have detected the breast masses, nor would they have come in for evaluation, and that could have led to an increased risk of them having advance staged breast cancer.

TIP

The key is to do regular self-breast exams to get familiar with your breasts and know what the normal feel of your breasts is, so you can identify when a lump or a change in your breasts occurs. If you do have a change in your breast, you must contact your doctor to have a breast evaluation. Don't ever take a change in your breast for granted.

What to Look For

REMEMBER

It's recommended that you check your breasts at least once a month, especially during the week after your menstrual period. If you're post menopausal, pregnant, or nursing, you should examine your breasts on the first day of the month. Breast tissue enlarges before and during your menstrual period due to hormonal changes and returns to normal afterwards. Examining your breast tissue when it is enlarged due to normal hormonal changes may lead to "false positives," whereby the person thinks they feel a new lump. If this lump regresses when hormone levels drop, it's not likely to be due to cancer.

Examining your breasts can take no more than ten minutes. When you examine your breasts, you're looking for the following things:

>> **Nipple direction:** Is there a change in the nipple direction? That is, has it changed, such as now appearing at an unusual angle, or is the nipple now turned inward (inverted) when it used to be the opposite?

>> **Nipple secretions:** Is discharge coming out of your nipple spontaneously (without stimulation or squeezing)? Is it milky, bloody, yellow, brown, or weeping (a slow discharge, or something like oozing out of a wound)?

>> **Areola changes:** Are there changes in the dark skin around the nipple? Is it swollen or puckering?

>> **Thickened skin:** Does the skin feel thicker? Thick tissue may be found in the upper or lower areas of heavy breasts, such as a bulge on the skin.

>> **Orange peel:** Do you have "orange peel" skin? This happens when the skin appears to have unusually large pores anywhere on the breast.

>> **Dimpling:** Is there new dimpling in the skin, or a sunken area?

>> **Swelling:** Is there swelling, above the breast or under the armpit?

Some of those changes may appear in a person's breasts normally or perhaps since puberty. It is most important to note the *new breast changes* that are different from prior breast changes. If you find any changes in your breast, notify your doctor. Breast changes that are found early are mostly treatable. Figure 4-1 illustrates.

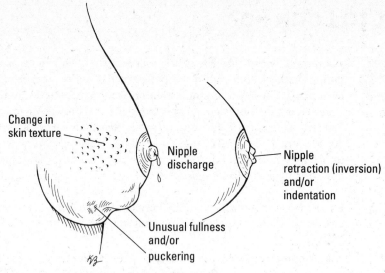

FIGURE 4-1: Some things to look for in your visual inspection.

Change in skin texture

Nipple discharge

Nipple retraction (inversion) and/or indentation

Unusual fullness and/or puckering

Illustration by Kathryn Born

Doing a Breast Self-Examination

As mentioned, there are a few different ways of examining your breasts. This section talks about three of the most common ways.

In the shower

Use the palm side of your hand to move gently over the breast and under the armpit in a circular motion and you may also need to "cup the breast" (four fingers on top side of breast and thumb underneath the breast) to feel the central portion of the breast. While doing your breast exam, apply light pressure to find changes just beneath the skin, medium pressure to feel changes further beneath the skin, and deeper pressure to feel changes close to the chest wall.

The wet skin will help your fingers to glide easier over the breast. You should check for thickness, lumps, and swelling.

In front of the mirror

>> **Hands on your side:** Place your arms at your side and look at your breast in the mirror. You can slowly rotate your upper body while your hands are at your side and flex your chest muscles.

>> **Hands on your head:** Raise your hands, place them on your head, and examine each breast for bulges or dimpling, especially underneath. It is normal to have dimpling on both breasts at the same location; if you only have dimpling on one breast, contact your doctor for an evaluation.

>> **Hands above your head:** Lift your hands above your head and look for breast changes, especially in the nipple area (such as inverted nipple).

>> **Hands on your hips:** Rest your hands on both hips and press firmly while you flex your shoulders backward. This position will allow you to flex your chest muscles while you rotate your upper body to look for changes in shape or appearance.

While lying down

Place a pillow under your mid-back. This allows your chest to expand. Then place your right hand behind your head and with your left palm and fingers press gently in small circular motions as if your breast is an imaginary clock.

TIP

Be systematic in how you do your breast exam. Start at the outside edges of your breast at the 12 o'clock position of the imaginary clock and move clockwise until you return to 12 o'clock again. Move a little toward the center of the clock and repeat. Keep moving in a circular motion and inward until you reach the nipple. Switch hands and repeat for your other breast.

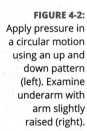

REMEMBER

At the end of the process, gently pinch each nipple between the thumb and the index finger to determine if there is any secretion. If there is, you must check with your doctor. Figures 4-2 and 4-3 illustrate a few self-exam techniques.

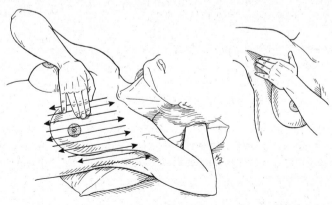

FIGURE 4-2: Apply pressure in a circular motion using an up and down pattern (left). Examine underarm with arm slightly raised (right).

Illustration by Kathryn Born

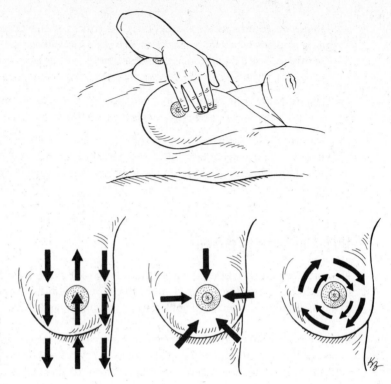

FIGURE 4-3:
Gently probe
each breast in
one of these
three patterns.

Breast Cancer Screening Guidelines

The purpose of breast cancer screening is, of course, early detection of breast cancer so you can get timely treatment if needed. The earlier anything is caught, the better. That's a no-brainer, right?

Unfortunately, some people run into psychological barriers. Some refuse to have a screening mammogram, for example, out of fear of the unknown, or they just don't want to know if they have cancer. Believe us when we say that, when it comes to cancer, ignorance is definitely *not* bliss.

Often individuals who avoid screening mammograms have already been through some earlier traumatic event. Some have had a close relative or friend who was diagnosed with breast cancer, and the progress of their disease has left a traumatized memory.

Screening is one thing you can do to be proactive about maintaining good health. We all may be diagnosed with a disease at least once in our lifetime but the disease does *not* have to be the cause of our death. Many who find out they have advanced breast cancer say in hindsight, "I wish I had gotten my mammogram every year," or, "I wish I'd had my doctor check this lump on my breast two years ago," or even, "I wish I hadn't ignored the rash on my breast for nine months thinking it was eczema or dermatitis."

TIP

Don't let such regret happen to you. Make someone's *I wish* be your *I will*.

Traditionally, screening mammogram starts at age 40. In recent years there have been controversial changes with the screening guidelines across many organizations. Some recommend beginning screening at a later age (between 45–50 years of age), and some recommend screening every two years (instead of annually) or only when you have a life expectancy of ten years or more.

Table 4-1 shows some recent screening recommendations among some major medical organizations.

TABLE 4-1   ## Breast Cancer Screening Guidelines

	ACR 2010	ACBG 2011	ACS 2015	USPSTF 2016	AAFP 2016
Women 40–49 years w/avg risk	Screening with mammogram annually.	Screening with mammogram and complete a clinical breast exam with your doctor annually.	Women 40–44 can choose to start annual screening with mammograms. The risk of screening and potential benefits should be considered. Women 45–49 should get mammograms annually.	The decision to start having screening mammogram before age 50 is an individual one. If you have a higher value on the potential benefit than the potential harms, then you may begin screening every two years from ages 40–49.	The decision to start having screening mammogram is an individual one. If you have a higher value on the potential benefit than the potential harms, then you may begin screening.

(continued)

TABLE 4-1 *(continued)*

	ACR 2010	ACBG 2011	ACS 2015	USPSTF 2016	AAFP 2016
Women 50–74 years w/avg risk	Screening with mammogram annually.	Screening with mammogram and complete a clinical breast exam with your doctor annually.	Women 50–54 should get mammograms every year. 55+ should switch to having mammograms every two years, or have the choice to screen annually.	Screening mammogram every two years.	Screening mammogram every two years.
Women 75+ w/avg risk	Screening mammogram should stop when life expectancy is less than five to seven years on the basis of age and chronic medical conditions.	Women should talk with their doctor to decide whether or not to continue to have screening mammogram.	Screening should continue as long as the woman is in good health and is expected to live 10 or more years longer.	Current research is insufficient to assess the balance of benefits and harms of screening mammogram in women 75 years or older.	Current research is insufficient to assess the balance of benefits and harms of screening with mammography.
Women with dense breasts	In addition to screening mammogram, an ultrasound can be considered.	Insufficient evidence to recommend for or against breast MRI screening.	Insufficient evidence to recommend for or against breast MRI screening.	Current research is insufficient to assess the balance of benefits and harms of screening for breast cancer using ultrasound, breast MRI, or digital breast tomosynthesis (DBT) or other methods in women identified to have dense breasts on an otherwise negative screening mammogram.	Current evidence is insufficient to assess the balance of benefits and harms of screening for breast cancer using ultrasound, breast MRI, DBT, or other methods.

TIP

Breast specialists and clinicians feel strongly about their patients doing breast self-exams, getting clinical breast exams, and completing screening mammograms. The USPSTF recommendations in Table 4-1 do not come from a breast specialist who takes care of newly diagnosed breast cancer patients on a daily basis. Countless times we (your authors, who are breast cancer specialists) have had patients who come to see us with a complaint of a breast mass that they or their spouse has felt.

The organizations listed in Table 4-1 could not agree on the breast cancer screening guidelines. What *is* agreed upon is that you should start screening between 40–50 years of age. Talk with your doctor or healthcare provider to determine your risk for breast cancer and discuss whether you should have a mammogram. Therefore, you have to make an informed decision about your mammogram screening that is best for you, taking into consideration your family history, environmental exposures, health behaviors, and age.

Mammograms: The Go-to Tool

A *mammogram* (see Figure 4-4) is a procedure done with a machine that takes an X-ray of the breast. Mammograms can help to find breast cancer early, sometimes up to three years before a mass can be felt. Well-developed breast cancers are almost always seen on a mammogram, but cancers that are not as developed can be missed on a mammogram.

Sometimes your mammogram may show small areas of calcium in patterns within the breast called *calcifications*, and these are often present in the breast with no lump. Calcifications can sometimes mark areas of the breast that might develop into cancer or they can be present in noncancerous changes in the breasts. The skill and expertise of a good radiologist is necessary to read the different calcium patterns and determine which change is most likely related to cancer.

Tomosynthesis (tomo) mammogram

Currently the *tomo* mammogram (sometimes called a *3D* mammogram, depending on manufacturer) is the best type of mammogram for screening. A conventional mammogram takes images of the breast in four views, whereas a tomo mammogram takes images and divides them into an average of 40 slices or more, depending on the size of the breast. Tomo mammograms help the radiologist find breast cancers earlier — even many *years* earlier than the conventional mammogram would have found it. Tomo mammograms also help reduce the number of patients that are called back for additional imaging involving overlapping tissues or dense breasts.

TIP

Research has shown that tomo mammograms detect 30 percent more breast cancers and reduce the callbacks for additional imaging by 40 percent. Radiologists feel that the tomo mammogram is so useful that almost every patient should want to have it.

One drawback to tomo mammograms is that they aren't available at every mammography center. And they may cost more than conventional mammograms. Although some insurance carriers may not cover the cost for 3D tomo mammograms, when you add up the costs of a regular screening mammogram and a breast ultrasound, that usually costs much more than a tomo mammogram, a diagnostic (or call back) mammogram, and a breast ultrasound.

REMEMBER

Some cancers don't show clear signs on a mammogram. So always tell your doctor if you find any lump or changes in your breast, even if you recently had a mammogram. Mammograms have saved countless lives, but they're not perfect. There is no screening test that will detect cancers 100 percent of the time. Unfortunately, there will always be some breast cancers that will be missed or not seen on a mammogram. However, tomo mammograms detect more cancers at an earlier phase of development.

Advantages of screening mammograms

Most experts will argue that the benefit of the screening mammogram in identifying breast cancer early far outweighs the risk of not having it done:

>> The earlier a change in your breast is identified, the better your chances.

>> Being diagnosed with breast cancer at an early stage makes you less likely to need a mastectomy (whole breast removal) or chemotherapy.

We do know that research has shown that women 50–69 derive the most benefit from screening mammograms. However, one inherent flaw with any research finding is that they can only report on a targeted group of women who voluntarily participate in a screening study. For example, the research may have been done only on one or two specific ethnic groups of women (such as Asian or Caucasian) aged 50 and older. Can those results be applied to African American or Latin American females, or to women under age 40? These are the questions you must wrestle with as you make the decision to start having screening mammograms.

Disadvantages of screening mammograms

Conventional mammograms are still useful, but a breast ultrasound may be needed in patients with dense breast or high risk. And as helpful as mammograms have been, there are a few downsides.

Overdiagnosis

Even though getting regular screening mammograms reduces the risk of dying from breast cancer, there is still some risk. Women who get regular screening mammograms may still get diagnosed with breast cancer and may also die from the disease. The most common risk of getting screening mammograms is that they may show early cancers that, if they had remained undetected, may not have caused any symptoms or become life-threatening. Ductal carcinoma in situ (DCIS) — small, invasive breast cancers that would have never caused a problem — are often overdiagnosed. These breast cancers often stay the same size or even shrink on their own. Often the person may die from another cause instead of from breast cancer. Overdiagnosis may cause you to have unnecessary extra tests and treatment.

Overtreatment

Older studies done in the 1980s indicated that 40–50 percent of the time, DCIS can progress to invasive breast cancer. Recent research indicates fewer cases of DCIS progression.

It's difficult to tell which type of DCIS will become invasive breast cancer. The lower the grade of DCIS, the less likely it is to become invasive, whereas the higher the grade of DCIS, the more likely it is to become invasive. Because the prediction of DCIS severity is difficult, the overall recommendation is to remove the DCIS tumor in healthy patients. Typical treatment for DCIS is with lumpectomy (breast-conserving surgery) in addition to radiation therapy, mastectomy, or endocrine/hormonal therapy.

False positives and unnecessary follow-up tests

A mammogram may show *false positive* results — changes that are suspicious for breast cancer are seen on X-ray, but a biopsy turns up negative for cancer. Sometimes a mammogram shows a mass or change that requires you to keep following up at six-month intervals with no change. In addition to having more than one mammogram per year, you may be called for a diagnostic mammogram, breast ultrasound, breast MRI, or even a biopsy — with a final report showing negative for breast cancer. Even though a breast biopsy is generally a low-risk, safe procedure, there may be complications, such as bleeding or infection. Many changes in the breast such as a mass or calcifications are not breast cancer but can indicate other breast conditions, such as fibroadenoma, cyst, papilloma, and so on.

How a mammogram is done

The technologist at the image center will ask you to stand in front of a mammogram machine with two clear plastic plates. Your breast will be placed on one plate and the other plastic plate will firmly press your breast from above. The plastic plates will flatten the breast, and you must hold still while the X-ray is being taken (see Figure 4-4). You will feel some pressure on the breast. The technologist will repeat the process to take a side view of the breast and the other breast so they can be X-rayed in the same way. You may have a brief wait while the technologist checks to ensure that the X-rays show a good image of the breast and do not need to be redone.

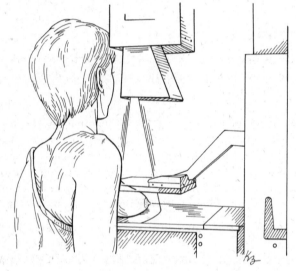

FIGURE 4-4: In a mammogram, the breast is flattened to enhance the X-ray image.

REMEMBER

The technologist can't tell you the results. Your X-rays will be read by a radiologist — a medical doctor specialized in diagnosing and treating diseases and injuries using medical imaging techniques, such as X-rays, ultrasound, magnetic resonance imaging (MRI), and more. A radiologist is the only person to provide you with the results of your mammogram.

Note: Your mammogram X-ray will look different from someone else's because, as we've emphasized, every breast is different. Some breasts are dense, fatty, or fibroglandular (discussed in the next section).

MAMMOGRAM SCREENING BEFORE 40

Sometimes it's necessary for you to start having screening mammograms under the age of 40. If you have a first-degree relative, such as a mother, father, sister, or brother, who developed breast cancer before the age of 50, then your screening should start 10 years earlier than the age they were diagnosed. Note the mention of father and brother, because men do get breast cancer. For most women under 40, you should discuss with your doctor when to start having screening mammograms.

Other Screening Tests: MRI and Ultrasound

Magnetic resonance imaging (MRI) of the breast — or breast MRI — is a test used to detect breast cancers and other changes in the breast. The breast MRI takes multiple pictures of your breast and combines them using a computer to provide more detailed images.

MRI has been used to find some breast cancers not seen on mammogram, but it is most likely to find a change in the breast that is not cancer (a false positive). To ensure that you verify the false-positive findings, you must do more tests and/or biopsies for resolution. This is why MRI is not normally recommended as a screening test for women at average risk of breast cancer, because it often means unneeded biopsies and other tests for many of these women. Figure 4-5 illustrates a breast MRI procedure.

A breast MRI is often used for screening of women who have a high risk for breast cancer or who have a known breast cancer gene mutation (such as BRCA1 or BRCA 2).

Breast MRI is also used after a breast biopsy returns a positive result for cancer and you are considering a lumpectomy. The breast MRI will show if there are additional cancers, if your cancer has extended or involves a larger area of the breast, and if there are additional cancers or in another location of the same breast or the other (contralateral) breast.

Ultrasound, sometimes called *sonography*, is an imaging technique that uses high-frequency sound waves that pass into the breast and bounce back from the breast tissue to form an image of the breast. You've probably at least seen ultrasounds done on TV and in movies with pregnant women. It involves the use of a small probe (*transducer*) on the skin that is lubricated with gel, and the sound waves form an image on the computer screen. Ultrasound is not a first-line screening tool for breast cancer, but it can be a helpful tool to examine masses that have been felt in the breast.

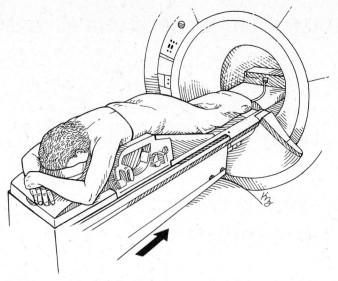

FIGURE 4-5:
Breast MRI
procedure.

Illustration by Kathryn Born

Ultrasound is harmless and doesn't use ionizing radiation. It's often used to diagnose breast abnormalities that may or may not be detected by physical exam, including the following:

>> Breast lump (benign or cancerous)

>> Bloody or spontaneous clear nipple discharge

>> Breast abscess

Ultrasound can show if a mass is a cyst (fluid-filled) or if it is solid (a noncancerous or cancerous tumor). Ultrasound can also show whether a mass has blood supply through it, which is more suspicious for a cancer.

Ultrasound is also used to examine the axillary lymph nodes or armpit lymph nodes for changes that may signify that an active disease is present in the breast or under the armpit. The axillary lymph nodes can become swollen if you cut your arm while shaving, develop an abscess or infection in the breast or armpit, or develop a breast cancer or lymphoma.

Ultrasound is also used to evaluate dense breasts. When a breast is dense with fibrous and glandular tissue, identifying a breast cancer on a mammogram can be more difficult — both dense breast tissue and breast cancer appear white on a mammogram. Ultrasound of the breast is also used to examine a breast mass in a pregnant woman, because a mammogram during pregnancy isn't recommended (due to exposure of radiation during imaging).

Using breast ultrasound as an addition to a screening mammogram has its pros and cons. The pros are that it provides a full examination of the breast and it can determine the type of breast mass, which ultimately can help to provide you with a diagnosis. The cons are that the ultrasound may show abnormal changes that were not seen on the mammogram, and multiple biopsies may be required — with a final diagnosis that is negative for breast cancer.

All in all, it is better to be safe. Ask yourself: What are you willing to do to ensure your breast health?

REMEMBER

If you have concerns about additional screening with breast ultrasound, you should discuss with your doctor to determine if it is right for you.

Chapter **5**

Understanding Breast Biopsies

Diagnostic images of the breast (mammograms, ultrasounds, and MRIs — refer to Chapter 4 for more) are like radar screens indicating the presence of an unidentified object. The images tell your doctor that something abnormal is in the area, but they don't indicate what the abnormality is. Like a pilot who is unsure of whether the radar is showing an airplane, a weather balloon, or an alien spaceship, your doctor needs additional information to determine whether diagnostic imaging shows a cancerous growth or something less serious. After all, most breast abnormalities are noncancerous.

The only way to know for sure the identity of any abnormality is to perform a breast *biopsy* — a medical procedure that involves extracting tiny samples of breast tissue and analyzing them for the presence or absence of cancerous cells.

Although we certainly don't expect you to look forward to your biopsy with eager anticipation, we do want you to fully understand the key role it plays in arriving at an accurate diagnosis, deciding whether treatment is necessary, and evaluating treatment options. We also want you to know what the procedure entails and how to make sense of the biopsy report. This chapter offers all that and more.

REMEMBER

A popular myth surrounding breast biopsies is that if cancer is present, the biopsy can cause the cancer to spread. This is *false*. Breast biopsies do not cause breast cancer (if present) to spread.

REMEMBER

If your doctor orders a breast biopsy, don't jump to the conclusion that your doctor thinks you have breast cancer. Your doctor is merely gathering additional information to make a well-informed diagnosis.

A biopsy is more likely to detect one of the following less serious conditions:

>> **Dense breast tissue:** Dense breast tissue appears white on mammograms and can easily be mistaken for an abnormal growth. Breast tissue density varies among women, and individuals may have areas of breast tissue that are denser than other areas. Dense breast tissue can make it difficult to detect tumors and other abnormalities through diagnostic imaging.

>> **Fibrocystic breast disease:** This is very common in women aged 20–50 and less common in postmenopausal women, unless they are taking hormone replacement therapy. This condition is related to hormonal changes and may increase just prior to your menstrual cycle or if you consume more caffeine than usual. Fibrocystic breast disease consists of breast lumps or areas of lumpiness or thickening that tend to blend into the normal surrounding breast tissue. An affected breast will feel firm and contain breast *cysts* (fluid-filled sacs), which may make the breast feel larger, lumpy, tender, or may cause dark brown or green non-bloody nipple discharge that tends to leak without pressure or squeezing nipple discharge or persistent pain.

>> **Benign (noncancerous) breast tumors:** A *benign* tumor is a mass of cells that have grown faster and thicker than normal. They may hurt, but benign tumor cells don't spread, and they're not dangerous. However, some benign breast tumors, such as those classified as atypical hyperplasia and papilloma, can increase your *risk* of developing breast cancer. (For more about tumors, see "Making Sense of Your Biopsy Results," later in this chapter.)

>> **Breast calcifications:** Calcium salts may gather within the breast and appear as white spots on mammograms. Calcifications are common and usually harmless. You probably won't feel them, and they don't cause any pain or discomfort. Sometimes calcifications can become harmful when they start clustering together.

Knowing What a Breast Biopsy Entails

To perform a breast biopsy, your doctor (usually a radiologist or surgeon) uses a needle or scalpel to remove small tissue samples from inside the breast, from the skin of the breast, or from axillary (under the armpit) lymph nodes. (For additional details about the procedure, see "Knowing what to expect on the day of your biopsy," later in this chapter.)

Tissue samples are taken from multiple areas of the mass or suspicious area of the breast or underarm to increase the probability of getting cancer cells (if present) within the sample. Even though multiple tissue samples are collected at the suspicious site, they are referred to collectively as *the biopsy.*

These tissue samples (called *cores*) are sent to a pathologist for analysis. (A *pathologist* is a doctor who specializes in examining cells under a microscope to identify the presence or absence of disease.)

You can expect to wait one to seven days to receive the results. Time varies according to the availability of a pathologist, the distance of the pathologist from the site where the biopsy is performed, and the nature of the tests your doctor ordered. (For more about the results of a breast biopsy, see "Making Sense of Your Biopsy Results," later in this chapter.)

Getting the Right Type of Breast Biopsy

All breast biopsies involve the removal of breast tissue. However, the procedure varies in terms of the instruments and procedures used to perform it. For example, a *core needle* biopsy involves the use of a thin needle to extract a tissue sample about the size of a grain of rice, whereas a *surgical* biopsy involves the use of a scalpel to cut a larger piece of breast tissue out. In either case, the doctor will first use a smaller needle to numb up the skin around the biopsy site to help minimize any discomfort or pain. For most biopsy procedures, you will usually be awake, with the exception of a surgical biopsy. Procedures also vary in the digital imaging technology used to guide the doctor to the area from which the sample is to be taken.

Your doctor chooses the type of breast biopsy that will deliver the most accurate and useful results based on conditions detected in previous diagnostic examinations, as shown in Table 5-1.

TABLE 5-1   Choosing a Breast Biopsy Type

Condition	Breast biopsy type	Description
Mass detected via mammogram or ultrasound	Ultrasound-guided core needle biopsy.	A thin, hollow needle is injected into the mass under the guidance of ultrasound, to collect one or more samples.
Abnormal calcifications appearing as white spots on mammogram but that can't be felt	Stereotactic biopsy (you can have this procedure done in sitting position or lying face down, depending on the type of machine).	Breast tissue samples of the abnormal area are taken under the guidance of mammogram images.
Lesion (area of abnormal tissue) or abnormal breast finding only seen on MRI	MRI-guided core needle biopsy.	Breast tissue samples of the abnormal area are taken under the guidance of a breast MRI.
Suspicious lump in breast or under arm that can be felt during a clinical breast exam	Fine needle aspiration biopsy (ultrasound-guided core biopsy is often preferred because more tissue is collected to get a definitive diagnosis).	A very fine needle is attached to a syringe and a small amount of tissue and sometimes fluid is withdrawn from the lump (see Figure 5-1). Useful for distinguishing between a fluid-filled cyst and a solid mass.
Blisters or ulcerated skin on the breast	Skin-punch biopsy.	A circular tool is used to remove a small section of the skin and deeper layers of the breast tissue.
Breast mass or lesion in area difficult to access but seen on ultrasound, MRI	Surgical (open) biopsy may be *incisional* (to remove tissue samples for testing) or *excisional* (to remove the entire mass, as in a lumpectomy). This procedure is less used because the ultrasound-guided biopsy, MRI-guided biopsy, and stereotactic biopsy are attempted prior to deciding on surgical biopsy.	Breast or general surgeon surgically removes the mass or suspicious area of the breast. This involves giving you sedation or *general anesthesia* (that is, being "put to sleep").
Used for abnormal lesion(s) visualized only on tomosynthesis mammography	Tomosynthesis-guided biopsy (the machine is upright and is often added to existing equipment such as machine for stereotactic biopsy).	The breast that is being biopsied will be compressed (similar to a mammogram), while tomo mammographic technique is used to locate the abnormality. The radiologist injects a local anesthetic such as Lidocaine into the skin and deeper tissues to numb the area. A very small skin incision is made. The abnormality will be located by tomo, and several tissue samples will be extracted and sent to the pathologist for interpretation.

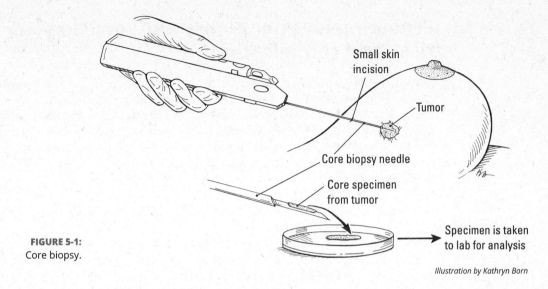

FIGURE 5-1:
Core biopsy.

If your doctor ordered a stereotactic or MRI-guided core needle biopsy, the proce-dure may strike you as a little odd. With a stereotactic biopsy, you lie face down on a table with your soon-to-be-biopsied breast extending down through a hole in the table. Your breast is squeezed between two mammogram plates, and X-rays are taken to show the doctor where to poke the needle.

The MRI-guided core needle biopsy is similar, but your breasts nestle in a depres-sion in the table. Although it sounds like something out of the Middle Ages, your doctor *is* performing a modern medical procedure.

Playing an Active Role in Your Breast Biopsy: Before, During, and After

Medical outcomes are always better when the patient plays an active role. The same holds true for a breast biopsy. When you know what to expect before, during, and after the procedure, you're likely to be less anxious and take the steps neces-sary to reduce risks, improve recovery, and follow up on results. This section discusses how to play an active role in your breast biopsy.

Preparing for your biopsy and reducing risks and complications

Soon after your biopsy is scheduled, the doctor who will perform it (a radiologist or breast surgeon) should inform you of the type of biopsy you will have. They should explain why it was chosen, discuss the benefits and risks, and briefly describe the procedure. You may receive a packet that includes a description of the procedure and instructions explaining what to do to prepare for the procedure (such as stop taking certain medications and arrange for someone to drive you home afterward).

TIP

If you have any questions at all, don't hesitate to call the office and ask.

Biopsy risks are associated primarily with allergies or sensitivities to any medications used during the procedure, reactions to the general or local anesthetic, other health conditions you may have (such as diabetes), and other medications you take or substances you consume. Possible complications resulting from the procedure include bruising or pain, bleeding, hematoma (solid–like mass or swelling of clotted blood at the site within the tissues), infection, slow healing, or scarring.

Team up with your doctor to reduce risks:

>> Tell your doctor if you have any allergies, so your doctor knows to avoid using certain medications.

>> Tell your doctor if you are taking blood-thinning medications such as aspirin, warfarin, heparin, ibuprofen, or naproxen, because these medications may increase bleeding at the biopsy site. (To reduce bleeding, stop using these medications for seven days prior to the biopsy or as instructed by your doctor.)

>> Tell your doctor if you have a history of diabetes and whether you have good diabetes control. Poor diabetes control can delay wound healing at the biopsy site and increase the risk of infection. To improve your diabetes control you must take your prescribed medications (for example, tablets or insulin) as ordered, eat the recommended diabetic diet with reduced carbohydrates, exercise regularly, and test your blood glucose level with your glucose machine (glucometer) as recommended by your doctor.

>> Tell your doctor if you smoke tobacco products or products that contain nicotine (such as cigarettes, chew tobacco, electronic cigarettes, and so on). Nicotine reduces oxygen to the tissue and can cause delayed wound healing and increase the risk of infection. Your doctor may recommend that you stop smoking or cut down on the amount of tobacco you smoke for several days before and after the procedure.

>> Don't use lotion, powder, perfume, or deodorant under your arms or on your breast prior to the biopsy procedure because these products can show up on the imaging or cause local skin reactions when combined with the sterilizing agent used to clean the skin. For that reason, it is usually recommended the skin be clean and free of cosmetic products.

Knowing what to expect on the day of your biopsy

Familiarizing yourself with the breast biopsy procedure may alleviate your anxiety. This section leads you step-by-step through the procedure, starting from the time the doctor or one of the doctor's assistants retrieves you from the waiting room:

1. The doctor or doctor's assistant reviews the risks and benefits of the biopsy procedure and asks you to sign a consent form.

2. The doctor or assistant cleans and sterilizes the area of the skin where the needle will be inserted or the incision will be made.

3. You can expect to receive a local anesthetic to numb the area from which samples will be taken or a general anesthetic to "knock you out." The local anesthetic may cause a burning or stinging sensation when it goes in, but the pain won't last long. It's important to numb the area up first so the procedure will be more comfortable. (You're more likely to need a general anesthetic if you're undergoing a surgical biopsy.) You may also receive a sedative, so you'll feel groovy during the procedure.

4. You may be instructed to sit up or lie down on your back, on your side, or face down on a special table. Again, this varies depending on the type of biopsy. (Diagnostic imaging equipment may be used to help your doctor locate the tissue to be biopsied.)

5. The doctor performing the biopsy may need to make a very small incision to gain access to the tissue that needs to be biopsied. If you're having a surgical biopsy, a longer incision may be required.

6. The doctor inserts the needle into the tissue to be sampled, extracts a core sample, and places it in a preservative or formalin to be sent to the pathologist. (This step is repeated approximately three to five times to obtain additional samples.)

7. The doctor places a tiny metal or titanium clip at the biopsy site to mark it for future examination or surgery, if necessary. The clip will appear on diagnostic images, but you will probably not notice it. It's important to have this clip inserted because it provides a map to the site that was biopsied in the breast, should it need to be sampled again in the future.

A small percentage of patients don't want anything "left" in their bodies, as they feel this will cause them pain or harm. But having this spot marked with a clip is very helpful for future mammograms so that the area with the abnormality can be monitored over time (if it's not all surgically removed).

8. If an incision was made, the doctor closes it with sutures or adhesive strips and applies dressing. If no incision was made, the doctor applies pressure and possibly a cold compress to stop the bleeding and then dresses the puncture site.

9. To wrap things up, the assistant is likely to take you back to an observation area for several minutes to make sure you're doing okay before you're released. You may obtain oral or written instructions on how to care for the wound, when to schedule a follow-up visit, and when to expect the results.

TIP

If you're not told, ask when you can expect to receive the results, from whom the results will come (radiologist, surgeon, primary care physician, nurse practitioner), and in what form — phone call or in writing. If you have a preference for how you receive the results, let it be known; the medical center has its own procedures but may make an exception upon request.

Waiting for your biopsy results

After your biopsy, you can expect to wait for one to seven days to receive the results. The amount of time varies depending on several factors. The method of informing patients of their biopsy results also varies. With some medical centers, the radiologist or surgeon calls the patient directly. Others may send the results to the gynecologist or primary care physician, who then contacts the patient to discuss the results. And some medical centers mail the results to the patient. Regardless of who the messenger is and in what form the message arrives, the results can be a source of relief or grief.

If you have a preference for how you're contacted and by whom, tell someone in charge of such things at the medical center. Most people (women and men alike) prefer to receive good news as soon as possible and welcome the opportunity to receive the good news over the phone. Many of these same people, however, would rather receive bad news (results that show cancer) in person from their doctor, who can explain the results and discuss next steps.

REMEMBER

Always request a copy of the biopsy report so you can keep it in your medical file. Having a copy of your report avoids delays in obtaining a copy in the future if another doctor needs to look at it or if you need to refer to the results later or share the results with family members.

Making Sense of Your Biopsy Results

You may receive your biopsy results in two forms: a cursory report, typically in the form of a letter, indicating whether or not the biopsy detected cancer, and the pathologist's report, which goes into much greater detail. This section aims to help bring you up to speed on some medical terminology that you may encounter as you read the results. It covers how to interpret breast biopsy reports (cursory and in-depth) and provides additional guidance on how to discuss the results with your doctor.

Grasping some basic medical terminology

As you read the biopsy results, you are likely to come across some unfamiliar terminology. Here are a few of the more common terms and their definitions:

>> **Atypical:** Abnormal/unusual, but not cancerous. However, surgery is recommended for atypical lesions found on core biopsy.

>> **Benign:** Noncancerous and unlikely to spread.

>> **Carcinoma:** Cancer that started with cells that line organs, called *epithelial* cells. This can be invasive or infiltrating or *in situ* (see upcoming definition).

>> **Hyperplasia:** More cells than normal in a tissue sample. There are several types of hyperplasia:

- **Usual ductal hyperplasia (UDH):** The pattern of cells is very close to that of normal cells.

- **Atypical ductal hyperplasia (ADH):** The presence of more cells than normal and cells with an unusual appearance in the lining of the ducts.

- **Atypical lobular hyperplasia (ALH):** The presence of more cells than normal and cells with an unusual appearance in the *lobules* (lobes of glandular tissue in the breast are further subdivided into lobules that produce milk — Chapter 1 talks more about lobules).

>> **In situ:** Latin for "in place," meaning the cancer has not spread. There are two types of in situ:

- **Ductal carcinoma in situ (DCIS):** This is a breast cancer. (Read more about DCIS in the section "Most common types of breast cancer.")

- **Lobular carcinoma in situ (LCIS):** This *is not* cancer. It is formed from abnormal cells in the lobules or milk ducts of the breast. When you're diagnosed with LCIS, however, you *are* at an increased risk for developing breast cancer in the future.

» **Invasive or infiltrating:** Cancer has spread or is likely to spread from its site of origin to nearby tissue.

» **Malignant:** Cancerous, has or is likely to spread.

» **Negative:** Is absent (not present).

» **Neoplasia:** Uncontrolled cell growth, may be benign or cancerous.

» **Noninvasive:** Cancer has not spread at this time.

» **Positive:** Is present.

» **Sarcoma:** Cancer that started with cells that don't line organs, called *parenchymal* cells.

These are just a few of the medical terms you're likely to encounter in a biopsy report. The following sections include other terminology you may see.

Sorting out the nuances of "abnormal"

Instead of *negative* and *positive*, some reports use *normal* and *abnormal* to indicate the condition of the cells that the pathologist examined. As you might expect, normal is all good — the tissue that was biopsied is normal tissue with no sign of cancer. Abnormal means that the cells are unusual (atypical) but they may be cancerous or noncancerous.

If your report shows that a tissue sample was abnormal without cancerous cells, you may have a benign tumor or some other tissue abnormality, such as one of the following:

» **Atypical ductal hyperplasia (ADH):** Having ADH increases your risk of developing breast cancer in the future, but these cells are not cancerous themselves.

» **Atypical lobular hyperplasia (ALH):** Having ALH increases your risk of developing breast cancer in the future, but these cells themselves are not cancerous.

» **Breast cyst:** Fluid-filled sac located inside the breast that is usually benign (not cancerous). You can have one or many breast cysts, and they can happen in one or both breasts. They can feel like a grape or fluid-filled balloon and may be tender at times.

» **Calcifications:** Very small calcium deposits that can develop in the breast tissue. They can appear like white dots or flecks on the mammogram image but can't be felt during a breast exam. Breast calcifications can have varying diagnosis. Some calcifications can be diagnosed as benign, DCIS, or IDC (read more about IDC in the section "Most common types of breast cancer").

» **Fibroadenoma:** Fibrous and glandular breast tissue. These often feel like smooth, rubbery lumps that may be painful.

» **Intraductal papilloma:** Wart-like growth in the milk duct of the breast usually close to the nipple, which may cause pain and nipple discharge.

» **Lobular carcinoma in situ (LCIS):** Having LCIS increases the risk of developing breast cancer (specifically DCIS or IDC) in the future.

» **Radial scar, or complex sclerosing lesion:** This is *not* a scar. It is an area of the breast tissue that has hardened. It's not felt but is often only found on a routine mammogram or during evaluation of breast symptoms.

If your report shows that a tissue sample was abnormal and contained cancerous cells, you have one of the types of breast cancer discussed in the next section.

Most common types of breast cancer

Here are the most common breast cancers:

» **Ductal carcinoma in situ (DCIS):** Noninvasive, DCIS starts in the ducts of the breast where milk passes through to the nipple. The cancer cells have not spread through the walls of the ducts in the surrounding breast tissue.

» **Invasive ductal carcinoma (IDC):** IDC starts in the ducts of the breast and spreads through the walls of the ducts in the surrounding breast tissue. If it continues to grow, it will then spread to the lymph nodes.

Less common types of breast cancer

These cancers are less common:

» **Angiosarcoma:** A type of cancer that starts in the cells that cover the blood vessels or lymph vessels. It occurs most frequently as a complication of previous radiation in the chest area.

» **Inflammatory breast cancer:** An aggressive breast cancer characterized by thick (like an orange peel) red skin that is warm to the touch.

» **Paget's disease of the nipple:** A type of cancer that starts in the duct and spreads to the nipple and then around the areola (the darker circle around the nipple). The skin of the nipple appears crusty, scaly, dry, and red, and may have areas of bleeding. The area around the nipple may burn and itch.

>> **Phyllodes:** A usually benign tumor that is large and bulky and grows quickly in the breast. In rare cases, it can be cancerous (malignant) and spread to other parts of the body.

TIP

If your biopsy report indicates the presence of cancer, ask to meet in person with your healthcare provider to ensure that you understand your biopsy results and your next steps.

Digging deeper into the pathology report when cancer is detected

If the biopsy results confirm the presence of breast cancer, the pathology report will contain results from additional tests that were done on the breast tissue biopsy sample. These results help indicate how fast the cancer may grow, how likely it is to spread to other parts of the body, how well certain treatments may work, and how likely the cancer will return after treatment.

These special tests include the following:

>> **Estrogen and progesterone receptor tests:** These tests measure the number of estrogen and progesterone hormone receptors in the breast tissue. Breast cancers that have these receptors are classified *estrogen-* or *progesterone-positive* (usually abbreviated ER+ or PR+) and can be treated with hormone therapy. Breast cancers that lack these receptors are estrogen- or progesterone-negative (ER–/PR–) and will not respond to hormone therapy. In general, cancers that are ER+/PR+ have a better *prognosis* (long-term outcome) than cancers that are negative for the receptors (ER–/PR–). Because estrogen and progesterone are involved in normal breast tissue growth, they can also lead to growth of cancerous breast tissue. Hormone therapy works to block the effects of estrogen and progesterone on the breast tissue.

>> **Human epidermal growth factor type 2 receptor (HER2/neu) test:** These tests measure the number of HER2/neu genes and the amount of HER2/neu protein in the breast tissue. If either level is unusually high, then the cancer is called *HER2/neu positive.* This type of cancer grows fast and is more likely to spread to other areas in the body. Importantly, there is a medication called Herceptin (generic: trastuzumab) that can inhibit this protein, which is why cancer specimens are tested for HER2 levels to help determine therapy.

More tests requested by a medical oncologist or breast surgeon can help determine whether chemotherapy will be beneficial in treatment.

Multigene tests measure the activity of genes within the tissue and may help predict the likelihood of the cancer spreading to other parts of the body or returning after treatment. The following multigene tests are often performed:

» **Oncotype DX 21:** This gene assay has two types of tests (from Genomic Health). The first, the Breast DCIS Score, measures risk of local recurrence. The other, the Breast Cancer Recurrence Score, predicts that a breast cancer recurrence score for early stage cancer (estrogen-receptor-positive, axillary-node-negative, or axillary-node-positive or HER2 negative in patients with one to three positive lymph nodes) will spread to other parts of the body. This score will help to predict whether receiving chemotherapy will give you any benefit for reducing your risk of cancer coming back. If the risk is high, chemotherapy may be recommended to lower the risk.

» **MammaPrint:** This 70-gene assay (from Avandia) is used to predict whether stage I or stage II axillary-lymph-node-negative breast cancer will spread to other parts of the body. If the risk is high, then chemotherapy may be recommended to lower the risk.

Based on the results of these special tests, your breast cancer may be described as any of the following:

» *Hormone-receptor-positive* means that the cancer is either estrogen-receptor positive or progesterone-receptor positive.

» *Hormone-receptor-negative* means that the cancer is neither estrogen-receptor-positive nor progesterone-receptor-positive.

» *Estrogen-receptor-positive* (or ER+) means that the cancer cell has estrogen receptors on its surface, which suggests that the growth of the cancer was promoted by estrogen.

» *Progesterone-receptor-positive* (or PR+) means that the cancer cell has progesterone receptors on its surface, which suggests the growth of the cancer was promoted by progesterone.

» *HER2/neu* is one of the growth factor receptor proteins that is found on both normal or cancer cells.

» *HER2/neu receptors* send signals to the breast cells to grow normally. If there are too many HER2 receptors on the cell, they send more signals, thus causing the cells to grow too quickly. When HER2/neu is positive, it gives your oncologist another way to treat your breast cancer (see Chapters 10 and 13 for more).

» *Triple negative* (ER–, PR–, HER2/neu–) means that the cancer cell has no estrogen, progesterone, or HER2/neu receptors on its surface. This type of cancer has a worse prognosis (outcome) and generally requires more intensive treatment.

Discussing your pathology report

The best person to deliver your pathology result is the radiologist or surgeon who completed the biopsy, because they can best help you understand the results. The pathology results will be discussed with reference to your breast imaging and/or your symptoms. For example, if you have an initial complaint of bloody nipple discharge, were sent for a breast ultrasound, and a breast mass was found, a biopsy will be recommended. What if that breast biopsy returns a result of fibroadenoma (a benign mass)? The radiologist or surgeon knows that a fibroadenoma is not associated with bloody nipple discharge, so they are now driven to do further imaging to find the reason for the bloody nipple discharge.

REMEMBER

Your primary care provider or general practitioner is *not* the best person to give you your pathology result — because they don't know certain information that the radiologist or surgeon may know.

Understanding your biopsy results and the next steps to take is important. Next steps will vary, depending on whether the biopsy detected cancer or not.

Discussing next steps if cancer is found

If the pathology report indicates that the tissue sample contains cancerous cells, you need to know whether the cancer has or is likely to spread, how fast it will spread, what treatments are likely to be effective, and so on.

Ask these questions and jot down the doctor's answers for future reference:

>> Is the cancer invasive or noninvasive?

>> If it is noninvasive, can it become invasive in the future?

>> If it is invasive, how fast is it likely to spread?

>> What stage is the cancer?

>> Are additional tests necessary? If so, what tests do you recommend?

>> What treatments do you recommend? For example, your doctor may recommend hormone treatment, chemotherapy, or surgery. The pathology report will contain valuable information to help your doctor choose the most effective treatment(s).

The shades of your pathology result

Your pathology result may be defined in three areas: black, white, or gray:

>> **Black** is the result that confirms cancer.

>> **White** is the result that is *not* cancer (benign).

>> **Gray** is the result of an uncertain lesion or mass that can increase your risk of developing breast cancer in the future.

Table 5-2 breaks down these distinctions further.

TABLE 5-2   **Description of Black, White, and Gray Areas of Pathology Result**

Shade	Pathology Result	Treatment
Black area	DCIS	Cancer — must be removed by surgery.
	IDC	
	Inflammatory breast cancer	
	Phyllodes	
	Paget's disease	
	Angiosarcoma	
White area	Fibroadenoma	Not cancer — does not need to be removed or aspirated (cyst) unless it causes pain and discomfort.
	Cyst	
	UDH	
Gray area	ALH	Uncertain — may be benign but must be removed by surgery.
	ADH	
	LCIS	
	Papilloma	
	Radial scar or complex sclerosing lesion	

Following up when no cancer is found

If the pathology report rules out cancer, you can do the happy dance, but you may not be out of the woods just yet. Your doctor may schedule you for a follow-up mammogram, breast ultrasound, or breast MRI in six months for comparison or to document no change in the abnormal tissue.

In the meantime, continue with your regular breast self-examinations and contact your doctor immediately if you notice any changes in your breasts.

REMEMBER

Chapter **6**

Stages of Breast Cancer

When someone finds out they have breast cancer, the next thing they would like to know is that it is in the early stage. Detecting *early stage* breast cancer is most often achieved through regular screening mammograms. But screening isn't foolproof — it doesn't catch all cancers by the early stage.

Someone may have had a mammogram seven months prior that was negative for any suspicious masses or calcifications on the X-ray, yet a 3 cm mass has just been discovered in a breast that is confirmed to be breast cancer. Now the question is whether the breast cancer has spread to the lymph nodes under the armpit or to other parts of your body.

It is important to know as much about any cancer as possible as soon as possible for the following reasons:

» To estimate your *prognosis* — the likely course of the disease and the chances for recovery.

» To identify the stage of your cancer and identify any *clinical trials* — research investigations where you can volunteer to test new treatments to prevent, detect, treat, or manage various diseases or medical conditions.

» To communicate effectively about your disease. Your doctors understand your disease by using common terminology for evaluating the results of treatment as well as the results from clinical trials.

Testing to Determine Stages

The following types of tests help determine your stage of breast cancer:

>> **Medical history and physical exams:** These gather information about you in general, including other illnesses you may have (such as high blood pressure, blood disorder, and so on) and about your breast cancer. In addition, the specialist may ask you information about your family history and may ask for additional details about any family members who have had cancer. The specialist will examine your body by looking, feeling, and listening for any unusual signs or symptoms. The exam can often show the location and sometimes the size of the breast tumor or whether the tumor has spread to the lymph nodes under the armpit.

>> **Imaging studies:** These produce pictures of what is going on inside your body. Mammograms, MRIs, ultrasounds, CT scans, and PET scans are part of imaging studies that are used to show the location of breast cancer, the size of tumors, and whether the breast cancer has spread to other parts of the body. CT and PET scans are mostly used to look for disease outside of the breast in women with advanced disease or tumors that have a high risk of spreading to other parts of the body.

>> **Laboratory tests:** These include sampling of blood, urine, and other fluids from your body to obtain more information about your breast cancer and your body's functions. For example, the comprehensive metabolic panel (CMP) measures levels of the liver enzymes aspartate aminotransferase (AST) and alanine aminotransferase (ALT). If these are above the normal range, it indicates that the liver is not functioning well, and that may trigger your doctor to request additional imaging of the liver to determine whether the breast cancer has spread to the liver.

>> **Pathology:** This is the report from the biopsy with the information about tumor size, growth rate, type of breast cancer cells, grade of tumor, and whether estrogen, progesterone, and HER2/neu receptors are present.

Chapters 4 and 5 cover such tests in more detail.

Overview of Breast Cancer Staging

Ten women with the same kind of breast cancer may all be in very different stages. *Staging* of breast cancer is a classification system that looks at how large the cancer is and determines whether it has spread to other organs in the body.

Sometimes breast cancer remains solely in the breast, but sometimes it spreads under your armpit to your axillary lymph nodes, and perhaps beyond. Obviously, the more it spreads, the more dangerous it is.

The *grade* of the tumor is part of the pathology report. The pathologists grade the appearance of the tumor cells in comparison to normal breast tissue. Tumor cells that are only slightly abnormal and still retain some resemblance to normal breast cells are called well differentiated. *Well-differentiated* tumors generally have a better prognosis then poorly differentiated tumors. *Poorly differentiated* (also called *undifferentiated*) tumor cells have little resemblance to normal breast tissue cells.

The stage and the grade of your breast cancer are also important because they help your doctor determine the best treatment for you as well as to determine your prognosis. The particular treatment for breast cancer is often based on staging, grading, and the individual medical history of disease. For example, some older patients with multiple health problems can't tolerate certain chemotherapies and/or surgery, so their treatment must change due to their *co-morbidities,* or other health problems.

Here are a few common terms we will be using in this chapter:

>> **Local:** The tumor or cancer is located inside the breast.

>> **Regional:** The tumor has spread to the lymph nodes under the armpit or breast or there are large tumors that involve the breast skin.

>> **Distant:** Breast cancer cells have spread to other parts of the body such as lung, liver, brain, bone, and so on.

>> **Oncologist:** A doctor specializing in *oncology,* the study of tumors. The specialist may be a breast surgeon or general surgeon. They may biopsy a tumor in the breast, and if determined to be cancer, remove the tumor. A medical oncologist treats breast cancer using chemotherapy, endocrine therapy, or other therapies, such as targeted therapies.

Early

When you're told you have *early* or stage 1 breast cancer it means that your breast cancer has *not* spread beyond the breast to the lymph nodes under the armpit. Tumor cells typically move to the lymph nodes on the same side of the body as the affected breast. The early stage is certainly the best stage because it is the easiest to treat and gives you the best chance of being cured.

Locally advanced

If you are told that your breast cancer is *locally advanced* or *regional*, it means that the cancer has spread to the lymph nodes, but it has not spread to another part of the body beyond the lymph nodes. The tumor also has one or more of the following characteristics:

>> Larger than 5 cm in size

>> Growing through the skin or chest muscle

>> Present in the lymph nodes under the armpit, and the lymph nodes appear to be stuck to each other and nearby structures

Local recurrence

Local recurrence is the term used to describe when the same type of breast cancer has come back in the area of the breast that was previously treated.

Metastatic or secondary breast cancer

Metastatic breast cancer is also often called distant, advanced, secondary, or stage IV breast cancer (discussed in more detail later in this chapter). A simple way to describe secondary breast cancer is that the cancer has spread from its original site in the breast to other parts of the body. Sometimes secondary breast cancer means that multiple sites in the body require treatment at the same time.

REMEMBER

Breast cancer in the lymph nodes under the armpit *is not* secondary breast cancer.

Even though a cure for secondary cancer has not been found, new advances in medical treatment can control the spread of the cancer and stabilize the disease for many years. If you respond very well to this treatment, the cancer is often managed as a chronic disease such as *rheumatoid arthritis,* an autoimmune disease in which the body's immune system mistakenly attacks the joints, which creates inflammation, swelling, and pain in the joints, or *lupus,* a chronic autoimmune disease where the body's immune system attacks normal, healthy tissue causing inflammation, swelling, and damage to joints, skin, blood, heart, lungs, and kidneys. Metastatic cancer flares up from time to time and requires active treatment until the cancer is stabilized again.

OVERVIEW OF BREAST CANCER GRADING

You may hear about breast cancer grades. The *grade* of breast cancer refers to how the cells look under the microscope and how fast they're growing. There are three main grades of breast cancer:

- **Grade 1:** Low grade (slow growing, well differentiated)
- **Grade 2:** Intermediate grade (moderate growing, moderately differentiated)
- **Grade 3:** High grade (faster growing, poorly differentiated)

Deciphering the TNM Staging System

Staging is used for any type of cancer to measure how much cancer there might be and where it is located. The TNM staging system and grading of the cancer is used by specialists to determine the best treatment for your breast cancer, and it also helps them estimate your prognosis.

The TNM system is the most widely used staging system in the world. The system is maintained by the American Joint Committee on Cancer (AJCC) and the International Union for Cancer Control (UICC) and is updated every six to eight years to include new advances in understanding cancer.

TNM is an acronym:

>> **T stands for tumor:** It indicates the size of the tumor and is essential to determining the stages of breast cancer. It can only be determined from the imaging tests and surgical pathology report. The size of the whole tumor can't be determined from the biopsy (which samples a small piece of the tumor). Imaging and/or final surgical pathology (when the tumor is removed as a whole) is the only way to determine the T.

>> **N stands for nodes:** It indicates whether the cancer has spread to the regional lymph nodes.

>> **M stands for metastasis:** It indicates whether the tumor has spread beyond the lymph nodes to other organs, called *distant metastasis*.

Table 6-1 summarizes the values for T, N, and M and what they mean.

TABLE 6-1   How to Read the TNM Staging System

TX	The tumor can't be measured.
T0	There is *no* primary tumor found.
TIS	The breast cancer cells are only growing in superficial tissue and not in the deep tissues of the breast. This may also be called *in situ* breast cancer (hence, the IS).
T1, T2, T3, T4	The numbers after the T describe the size of the tumor in centimeters and/or how much the cancer has spread to nearby tissues. The higher the T number, the larger the tumor or the more it has spread into nearby tissues. T1 < 2 cm T2 = 2–5 cm T3 > 5 cm T4 = Any size with direct extension into chest wall or skin

NX	Regional lymph nodes can't be evaluated.
N0	The breast cancer has not spread to the regional lymph nodes.
N1, N2, N3	The breast cancer has spread to the regional lymph nodes (number of lymph nodes and/or extent of spread). The higher the N number, the more lymph node involvement.

MX	Distant metastasis can't be evaluated.
M0	No distant metastasis or the breast cancer has not spread beyond the lymph nodes under the armpit or to the lung, liver, brain, bone, or elsewhere.
M1	Distant metastasis is present.

TIP

The specialist takes your information after your full examination and puts it together in the TNM format to provide you with your clinical stage. For example, breast cancer classified as T3 N2 M0 refers to a large tumor that has spread to nearby lymph nodes but not to other parts of the body.

Let's break down another example. T2 N1 M0 means the following:

» A single tumor 2.1 to 5 cm across.

» There is evidence of spread to any the regional lymph nodes (axillary or mammary).

» No evidence of spread outside the breast.

REMEMBER

The TNM information is used to justify any additional tests and referrals to other specialists. It's also used to develop a treatment plan.

Understanding Breast Cancer Stages

In terms of breast cancer, the process is described in five broad stages, labeled 0 through IV. This section delves into detail on breast cancer stages.

Stage 0 (zero)

There are two types of breast cancer in this stage:

>> Ductal carcinoma in situ (DCIS)

>> Lobular carcinoma in situ (LCIS)

(Refer to Figure 1-2 in Chapter 1 to see an example of DCIS.)

Stage I

Stage I breast cancer is divided into two parts, A and B:

>> **Stage IA breast cancer:** The tumor is 2 cm or smaller and has not spread to the lymph nodes.

>> **Stage IB breast cancer:** Small microscopic breast cancer cells are either found in the lymph nodes close to the breast and either no tumor is found in the breast or the tumor is smaller than 2 cm.

Figure 6-1 illustrates both stage IA and stage IB.

Stage II

Stage II breast cancer is also divided into two parts, A and B:

>> **Stage IIA:** There is either no tumor or the tumor is 2 cm or less in the breast, and microscopic breast cancer cells are found in one to three lymph nodes under the armpit or in the lymph nodes close to the breastbone. Or there is a tumor between 2–5 cm with no positive lymph nodes. Figure 6-2 illustrates stage IIA breast cancer.

>> **Stage IIB:** The tumor in the breast is larger than 2 cm but smaller than 5 cm, and small areas of breast cancer cells are in the lymph nodes close to the breastbone. Or there is a tumor greater then 5 cm, with no positive lymph nodes. Figure 6-3 illustrates stage IIB breast cancer.

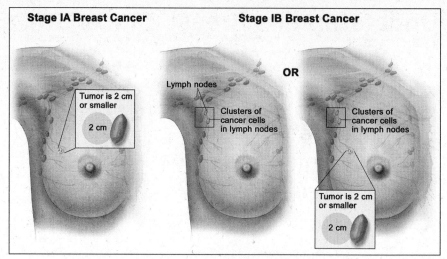

FIGURE 6-1:
Stage IA and
stage IB breast
cancer.

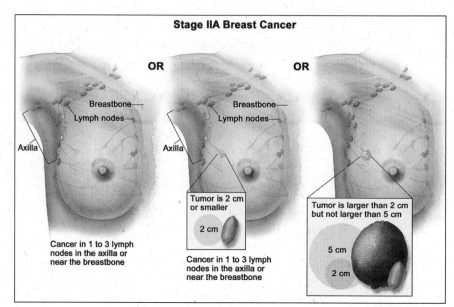

FIGURE 6-2:
Stage IIA breast
cancer.

Stage III

Stage III breast cancer is divided into three groups, A, B, and C:

>> **Stage IIIA:** No tumor is seen in the breast or the tumor is any size, and cancer is found in four to nine lymph nodes under the armpit or in the lymph nodes at the breastbone. Figure 6-4 illustrates stage IIIA breast cancer.

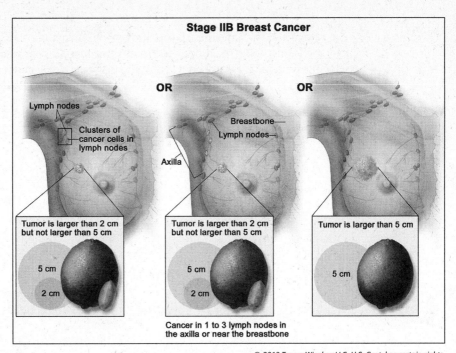

FIGURE 6-3:
Stage IIB breast cancer.

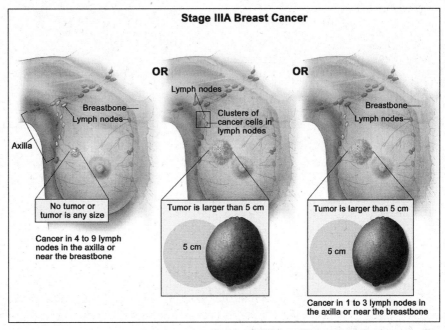

FIGURE 6-4:
Stage IIIA breast cancer.

>> **Stage IIIB:** The tumor has spread through the skin of the breast or the chest wall, and the skin has broken open and formed an ulcer or caused swelling. The cancer may have spread to no more than nine lymph nodes under the armpit or near the breastbone. Figure 6-5 illustrates stage IIIB breast cancer.

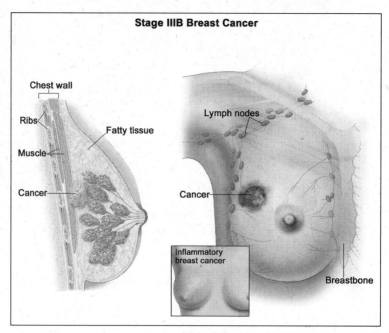

Stage IIIB Breast Cancer

Chest wall

Ribs

Muscle

Fatty tissue

Cancer

Lymph nodes

Cancer

Inflammatory breast cancer

Breastbone

© 2012 Terese Winslow LLC. U.S. Govt. has certain rights.

FIGURE 6-5:
Stage IIIB breast cancer.

REMEMBER

Breast cancer that has spread to the skin can also be diagnosed as inflammatory breast cancer.

>> **Stage IIIC:** The tumor is any size or there is no tumor. However, breast cancer has spread through the skin causing swelling or forming an ulcer and has spread to the chest wall. The breast cancer has also spread to at least ten lymph nodes in the armpit or near the breastbone. Figure 6-6 illustrates stage IIIC breast cancer.

Stage IV

Stage IV means that the tumor is any size, lymph nodes may or may not contain breast cancer cells, and the cancer has spread to other parts of the body such as the lungs, brain, liver, and/or bone.

Figure 6-7 illustrates stage IV breast cancer.

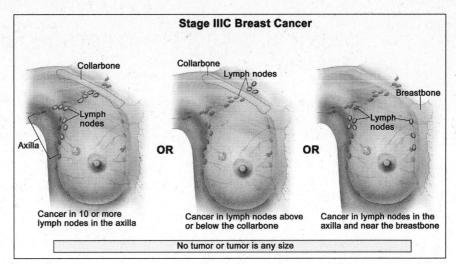

FIGURE 6-6:
Stage IIIC breast cancer.

Stage IIIC Breast Cancer

Collarbone

Lymph nodes

Axilla

Cancer in 10 or more lymph nodes in the axilla

OR

Collarbone

Lymph nodes

Cancer in lymph nodes above or below the collarbone

OR

Breastbone

Lymph nodes

Cancer in lymph nodes in the axilla and near the breastbone

No tumor or tumor is any size

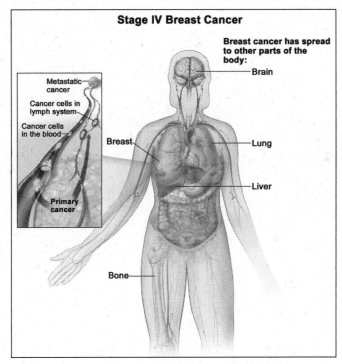

FIGURE 6-7:
Stage IV breast cancer.

Stage IV Breast Cancer

Breast cancer has spread to other parts of the body:

Brain

Metastatic cancer

Cancer cells in lymph system

Cancer cells in the blood

Breast

Lung

Liver

Primary cancer

Bone

CLINICAL STAGING AND PATHOLOGICAL STAGING

When breast cancer is diagnosed, the patient meets with a specialist who completes a physical exam, reviews any imaging tests (mammogram, X-rays, MRI) and biopsy results, and estimates the extent of cancer. This is called *clinical staging.* Clinical staging is used to help determine the best initial treatment for breast cancer and also serves as a baseline for comparison when determining how the cancer responds to treatment.

Pathologic staging is determined after the breast cancer and nearby lymph nodes are removed surgically. Surgery can be performed to take a tissue sample without removing the whole cancer to provide an accurate staging or surgery can be performed to remove the whole tumor and all the lymph nodes.

Sometimes on clinical exam the breast imaging and physical exams may show a breast cancer to be in an early stage, but after the surgery the tumor turned out to have been larger than previously predicted — or the breast cancer turned out to have spread to the lymph nodes under the armpit, even though prior to surgery the specialist had not detected it.

In other words, the clinical staging is a "guesstimation," and the only fully accurate description comes from the pathological staging at the end of surgery to remove the cancer. The lesson, unfortunately, is this: Don't get your heart set on what the specialist or doctor says is your stage prior to breast cancer treatment. Clinical staging is helpful for determining whether you should have surgery, chemotherapy, or hormonal therapy as the first treatment for your breast cancer. But the true stage of breast cancer will be determined at the end of surgery when you have your final pathology report, even if you have had *neoadjuvant* — treatment given as a first step to shrink the breast tumor before surgery is given — chemotherapy or hormonal therapy prior to surgery.

3

Treating Breast Cancer

Get an overview of all the major treatment options.

Find out about the different kinds of breast surgery and which one (if any) might be right for you.

Get informed about radiation therapy, how it works, and what to expect.

Check out everything you ever wanted to know about chemotherapy.

Get the lowdown on hormonal (endocrine), biological, and other cutting-edge treatments.

Stay on top of the latest innovations in breast reconstruction.

Find out about treatment options for advanced breast cancer.

Chapter **7**

Looking at Treatment Options

When a diagnosis of breast cancer happens, the mind immediately leaps to questions of treatment. If you get treatment for your breast cancer, what are your prospects? And can you be cured for good?

There's good news and bad news when it comes to treatment. One piece of good news is that there are many treatment options nowadays. Another piece of good news is that, if caught early, average breast cancer survival rates are actually pretty good. The "five-year survival rate" is often used when talking about prognosis in cancer. This number represents the percentage of people with that cancer who will be alive five years after their diagnosis. Five-year survival depends on which stage of cancer you have. If you combine all stages of breast cancer together, the survival rates are pretty good:

>> 5-year survival rate is 89 percent

>> 10-year rate is 83 percent

>> 15-year rate is 78 percent

When the breast cancer is located *only* in the breast, the 5-year survival rate can be as high as 99 percent, and approximately 61 percent of breast cancers are diagnosed at stage 1, or early stage. When the breast cancer has spread to the lymph nodes under the armpit, the 5-year survival rate falls slightly to 85 percent. The bad news is, of course, that things are worse if it has spread. If the breast cancer has spread beyond the lymph nodes under the armpit to the bones, liver, brain, or lung, then the 5-year survival rate drops to 26 percent.

Surviving breast cancer depends mostly on the stage of the cancer when you are diagnosed. Additional factors that can affect survival include the status (positive or negative) of your estrogen, progesterone, and HER2/neu receptors and whether the breast cancer is sensitive to specific medications. The *grade* of the breast cancer cells (how abnormal the cells are) can also be factored into calculating your prognosis.

REMEMBER

The prognosis of your cancer mostly depends on the stage of your breast cancer when it was diagnosed — including how large the tumor is and, most importantly, whether it has spread to other areas of your body.

Sometimes the cancer goes away but then comes back. If breast cancer is to come back, it usually occurs within the first three years. Some types of breast cancer are deemed to be *cured* if your cancer doesn't return within five years. Unfortunately, breast cancer can re-occur 10 or 20 years after you are diagnosed, although that is very uncommon. In general, the more time that passes since your initial breast cancer diagnosis, the less likely the breast cancer will return. Know that you *can* develop a new breast cancer in another location of the same breast or in the other breast.

Doctors may use one of the following tools to calculate your breast cancer outcome:

>> Nottingham Prognostic Indicator (NPI)

>> Adjuvant! Online

>> PREDICT

These tools use information about your stage, grade, and hormone receptors on your breast cancer cell to help calculate your outcome. Your doctors will choose the tool that is best for you, and the information will often help them to make decisions about the risk and benefits for specific treatments for breast cancer.

REMEMBER

Being diagnosed early and receiving timely treatment can significantly improve long-term survival of breast cancer.

But enough about prognosis and survival. Let's talk treatment. This chapter provides an overview of the main breast cancer treatment options, including surgery, chemotherapy, radiation therapy, and endocrine/hormone therapy, as well as targeted therapies using a multidisciplinary team approach to care. It also peeks at the idea of participating in clinical trials and the advantages of the new field of precision (personalized) medicine and how it relates to breast cancer. Once you have an idea of what the possibilities are, you can move on to the rest of the chapters in this part, which go into far greater detail for all these treatment options.

There are five main types of treatment for breast cancer:

>> Surgery

>> Radiation therapy

>> Chemotherapy

>> Hormone therapy or endocrine therapy

>> Targeted therapy or biological treatments

You may receive one type of treatment or a combination of several types of treatment, depending on your stage of breast cancer or other medical conditions. There is no one-size-fits-all when it comes to breast cancer treatment. The treatment for the cancer is determined from the pathology report and the person's age and general health, which, of course, can be different for each person.

Your doctor will review several factors before deciding which treatment is best for you. The most common factors include the following:

>> The *stage* (how large the cancer is and whether it has spread elsewhere in the body) of breast cancer

>> The *type* (for example, DCIS or invasive ductal carcinoma) of breast cancer

>> The *grade* (the appearance of the cancer cells and whether they are well differentiated or poorly differentiated) of your cancer cells

>> Whether or not you have gone through menopause

>> Whether your cancer cells have estrogen, progesterone, or HER2/neu receptors (sensitive to specific cancer drugs)

>> Your overall health, including any other illnesses, and whether they are managed

>> Your age, because older individuals with early breast cancer will likely never die of (or have symptoms) of their disease

You may have your own experiences with loved ones who have or have had cancer. Some of those experiences may be positive, and some may be negative. In addition, you may have specific preferences for what type of treatment *you* want for your breast cancer. It's important for you to discuss your preferences and personal experiences with your doctor concerning cancer treatment, so those preferences or questions can be answered or otherwise addressed. Scientists are always developing new treatments for cancer, and these treatments are always improving patients' prognoses. A treatment that a loved one may have received may not be the same treatment that your doctor is recommending for you — and even if it sounds the same, it may not work the same anymore. You must remain open-minded so that your doctor can inform you about all options and identify the pros and the cons to help you make an informed decision.

Surgery

Most individuals will begin their treatment with surgery. Your doctor may offer you several types of breast surgery and/or a choice about your treatment that is best suited for you. The type of surgery recommended will be based on what the pathology report says about, among other things, the size and location of the tumor.

This section briefly covers the main breast surgery options.

Lumpectomy or partial mastectomy (breast- conserving surgery)

In a lumpectomy, the lump is removed from the breast as well as a small surrounding area of normal tissue. That is, the entire breast is not removed. Lumpectomy is normally followed by several weeks of radiation therapy. Figure 7-1 illustrates the process of lumpectomy.

Mastectomy (total or simple)

This is probably what most people think of when they think of breast cancer surgery — removal of the entire breast. When the breast is removed, it is called a *total* or *simple* mastectomy. Figure 7-2 shows the result of mastectomy. Figure 7-3 illustrates a few of the possible techniques, each of which has positive and negative aspects.

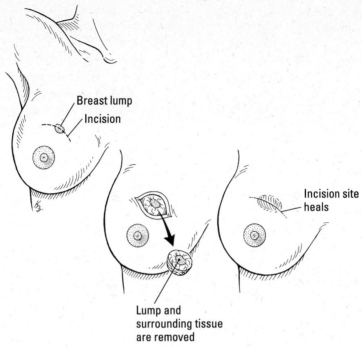

Breast lump
Incision

Incision site heals

Lump and
surrounding tissue
are removed

FIGURE 7-1:
Lumpectomy.

Illustration by Kathryn Born

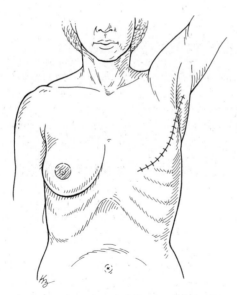

FIGURE 7-2:
After
mastectomy.

Illustration by Kathryn Born

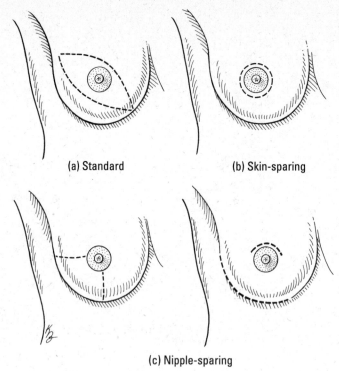

(a) Standard

(b) Skin-sparing

(c) Nipple-sparing

FIGURE 7-3:
Types of
mastectomy.

Illustration by Kathryn Born

Modified radical mastectomy

Modified radical mastectomy (Figure 7-4) is when the breast *and* lymph nodes under the arm are removed. If there are obvious signs or confirmed pathology (from biopsied lymph nodes under the armpit) that the cancer has spread to your lymph nodes, then a modified radical mastectomy can be performed.

Axillary lymph node dissection

This type of surgery involves opening the armpit (*axilla* or *axillary*) to examine or remove lymph nodes — small glands, part of the lymphatic system, that filter fluid from cells.

REMEMBER

Talk to your doctor more about this to determine the best treatment for you.

Axillary lymph nodes have three levels, shown in Figure 7-5:

>> Level I is the bottom level and located at the lower edge of the pectoralis minor muscle.

» Level II is located underneath the pectoralis minor muscle.

» Level III is located above the pectoralis minor muscle.

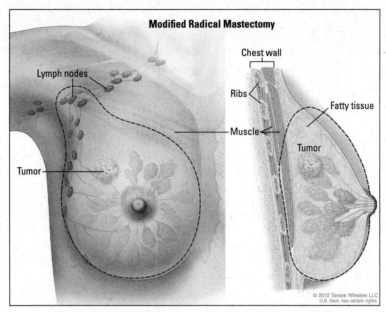

Modified Radical Mastectomy

Chest wall

Lymph nodes

Ribs

Fatty tissue

Muscle

Tumor

Tumor

© 2012 Terese Winslow LLC.
U.S. Govt. has certain rights

FIGURE 7-4:
Modified radical
mastectomy.

© 2012 Terese Winslow LLC. U.S. Govt. has certain rights

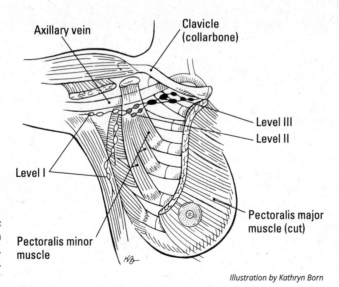

Axillary vein

Clavicle
(collarbone)

Level III
Level II

Level I

Pectoralis major
muscle (cut)

FIGURE 7-5:
Axillary lymph
nodes levels I, II,
and III.

Pectoralis minor
muscle

Illustration by Kathryn Born

Axillary lymph node dissection may be offered when the cancer has spread to your lymph nodes. However, recent studies have shown benefits of radiation of the lymph nodes instead of axillary dissection for select patients with minimal spread or micro metastasis (microscopic cancer cells) to the axillary lymph nodes and with T1 and T2 tumors (5 cm or less):

>> **Axillary lymph node dissection:** This usually involves the removal of lymph nodes in levels I and II, which can amount to approximately 5–30 lymph nodes. This procedure may be done at the same time with a mastectomy for women who have invasive breast cancer. It also can be done at the same time or after a lumpectomy. The total number of lymph nodes *involved* (showing evidence of cancer) is more important than the extent of cancer in any one node.

>> **Prophylactic mastectomy:** When a person chooses to remove one or both breasts pre-cancer, because of familial or genetic risk factors, or because of the possibility of re-occurrence of cancer.

>> **Sentinel lymph node biopsy:** The surgeon injects a blue dye and/or a radioactive dye below the nipple area several hours prior to surgery. The highest sensitivity for finding the sentinel node (the first draining lymph node of the breast) is when both dyes are used during the sentinel lymph node biopsy. During surgery the surgeon removes the tumor and is able to find a lymph node that has picked up the dye. The first lymph node to pick up the dye is called a *sentinel* lymph node. The dye will follow the same path that a tumor cell that breaks off from the main tumor would travel on its way to the lymph node. The dye creates a "trail of bread crumbs" for the surgeon to find the lymph nodes most likely to have tumor cells (that is, lymph node metastasis). See Figure 7-6.

Sentinel Lymph Node Biopsy

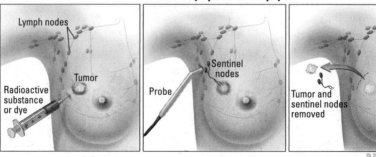

© 2010 Terese Winslow
U.S. Govt. has certain rights

FIGURE 7-6: Sentinel lymph node biopsy.

© 2010 Terese Winslow LLC. U.S. Govt. has certain rights

Chapter 8 goes into a lot more detail on breast cancer surgeries.

Breast Reconstruction

Breast reconstruction is when a surgeon rebuilds the breast using one of two main types of breast reconstruction: implant or your own tissue (tissue from belly, back, thigh, or buttock). Figure 7-7 illustrates sources of breast construction.

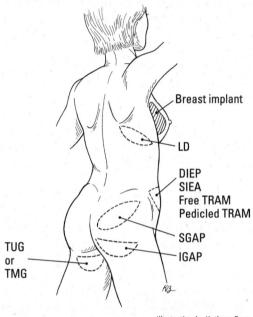

Breast implant

LD

DIEP
SIEA
Free TRAM
Pedicled TRAM

SGAP

IGAP

TUG
or
TMG

FIGURE 7-7:
Breast reconstruction options.

Illustration by Kathryn Born

As you can see, there are several surgical options for treating breast cancer, but it is your stage of breast cancer that determines which surgical options are best for you. Sometimes, based on the size of your tumor, your doctor may recommend a lumpectomy with or without a sentinel lymph node biopsy followed by several weeks of radiation (more on this shortly) with minimal change in the size of your breasts. But you may prefer to have the whole breast removed (mastectomy) and perhaps have a breast reconstruction. Regardless of what your doctor recommends and your preferences, here are some things you may find it helpful to consider as you decide among options:

>> How do you feel about having your whole breast removed?

>> How do you feel about having part of your breast removed?

>> How do you feel about having radiation therapy?

>> How quickly do you want your treatment to be completed?

>> How will you cope with travelling daily to get radiation therapy for several weeks?

>> Will you want to have immediate breast reconstruction or wait some months after surgery?

REMEMBER

There are no right or wrong answers to these questions — it is based on your values and preferences. Each woman is different and will approach their treatment decisions differently in a way that may be personal, social, financial, religious, or cultural.

WARNING

Some women may feel compelled to keep their breast and choose a lumpectomy even though that wasn't recommended by their surgeon because of the stage of their breast cancer. If you are that person, you should speak to your doctor or psychologist to help you determine why you are willing to put your life at risk by not getting the recommended type of surgery. In this case, a mastectomy would better ensure that all your cancer is removed and your risk of cancer coming back will be minimal.

If you feel strongly about not getting radiation, then lumpectomy should not be an option for you because you will not be receiving the standard treatment for your breast cancer. Mastectomy and possible breast reconstruction may be your only option in such a case, according to standard NCCN guidelines.

The type and timing of breast reconstruction may depend on your need for further treatment post–breast surgery, such as chemotherapy or radiotherapy. Breast reconstruction is optional — it's not required and won't change the outcome of the cancer.

TIP

Take the time you need to make the right decision after hearing all the options available to you for your treatment. Every decision you make may impact your survival positively or negatively. You can discuss your concerns with your doctor, family, and friends. Feel free to contact your breast specialist or nurse if you have additional questions before you make your treatment decision. Chapter 12 covers breast reconstruction in much more detail.

Radiation Therapy

Radiation, or *radiotherapy*, involves the use of a beam of high-energy rays to kill cancer cells in your breast or lymph nodes under your armpit or chest wall. Radiation therapy is usually recommended after a lumpectomy, when the breast cancer has spread to the lymph nodes under the armpit, or after a mastectomy and the surgical margins are still positive for cancer.

Side effects

Side effects from radiation can be *immediate* (also called *acute* or *early* side effects) or *long-term*, occurring after six months of radiation treatment.

Immediate side effects are typically related to skin reactions that may occur during radiation and may last for up to six months. If you are exposed to the sun a lot without wearing sunscreen, for example, you are more likely to get sunburn. Similarly, radiation will increase your risk of skin damage and other side effects that include the following:

>> Sunburn.

>> Darkening.

>> Tenderness and/or itching of the skin in the treatment area.

>> Peeling or flaking of the skin as treatment goes on, and this may result in a red, blistering, weepy skin reaction. Note that many individuals do not experience this symptom, and your radiation oncologist may provide you with special topical creams to use during radiation to reduce the risk of peeling and blisters from developing.

Side effects that may occur immediately and long-term

>> Pain in the breast or chest area in the form of aches, twinges, or sharp shooting pain

>> Swelling of the breast or chest

>> Stiffness or discomfort around the breast/chest or shoulder

>> Fatigue or tiredness

>> Hair loss under the armpit or chest area

>> Sore throat

>> Hardening of the tissue, known as fibrosis, caused by the accumulation of scar tissue

>> Dry cough or shortness of breath because of inflamed treatment area

Serious side effects that can occur later

» Weakening of the bones under the treated area, which can lead to rib and collarbone fractures

» Injury to the nerves in the arm, which may cause numbness, tingling, weakness, pain, and possible loss of movement

Immediate side effects usually occur around 10–14 days after starting radiation treatment, but can happen later in treatment or after it has finished.

The severity of your skin reactions depends on a few factors:

» Dose of radiation given

» Your skin type

» Existing skin conditions, such as eczema, psoriasis, and so on

TIP

If you have existing skin conditions, let your radiation oncologist/doctor know before starting treatment because it may be useful for you to meet with a dermatologist (skin specialist) for advice.

Skincare during radiation therapy

You must take special care of your skin that is being treated with radiation. Your radiation oncologist or radiation *technologist* (who administers the radiation therapy treatments) will provide you with specific skincare instructions at the center. Most instructions will include the following actions and precautions:

» Have a shower instead of a bath.

» Wash the treated area gently with warm water using a mild soap and pat the skin dry with a soft towel.

» Use a fragrance-free deodorant.

» Use a mild moisturizer or recommended topical cream to keep skin soft.

» If you want to use anything else on the skin in the treatment area, you must discuss this with your radiation doctor.

» Avoid exposing the treated area to extremes of temperature such as heat pads, saunas, or ice packs during radiation treatment.

» Avoid exposing the treated area to sun while having radiation and afterwards, until all skin changes at the treatment site have healed.

>> Avoid getting sunburn after treatment. Always use a sunscreen with a high *sun protection factor* (SPF) of 50 and above. You should also apply sunscreen under clothes because, thought it isn't widely known, it is possible to contract sunburn through clothing.

>> Avoid swimming during treatment and afterwards until all skin reactions have healed. Chemicals in the swimming pool may cause skin irritation, and a swimsuit can cause friction and discomfort at the treatment site.

>> Wear a soft cotton bra or vest during treatments to avoid rubbing or friction that can worsen skin reactions.

>> Avoid wearing underwire bras until your skin is healed.

Your radiation technologist will monitor your skin during treatments. When a skin reaction develops, they will advise you on caring for your skin.

WARNING

If you develop a skin reaction during radiation, it should heal within four weeks from the date of your last treatment. If your skin is taking longer than four weeks to heal, or you have severe blisters and skin peeling, you *must contact* your radiation treatment team or breast care nurse for advice.

Chapter 9 talks about radiation therapy in a lot more detail.

Chemotherapy

Chemotherapy involves administration of drugs that kill the rapidly dividing cells in the body — the cancer cells. Sometimes chemotherapy is given as a single medication or it can be a combination of medications. Combination medications are given to increase the chance of killing many different cells involved in your breast cancer.

Chemotherapy can also cause injury to healthy cells, thus increasing your risk of unwanted side effects, including the following:

>> Acid reflux

>> Anemia

>> Change in appetite

>> Change in tastes

>> Changes in blood circulation

>> Diarrhea

>> Fatigue

>> Hair loss

>> Nerve injury

>> Stomach pains

Check out Chapter 10 for more in-depth information on chemotherapy.

Endocrine or Hormonal Therapy

Endocrine or *hormonal* therapy is used to reduce the risk of breast cancer coming back or to reduce the risk of breast cancer developing in an individual with no prior diagnosis of breast cancer. Check out Chapter 11 to find out how endocrine therapy is used as initial treatment for breast cancer, post treatment after breast cancer surgery, and for prevention of breast cancer in individuals at risk for breast cancer.

Targeted Therapy: Herceptin and Others

Targeted therapy is also called *biological* therapy. It affects specific protein-receptor targets (called *biomarkers*) found only on cancer cells. These protein-receptor targets are responsible for the growth and spread of cancer cells. Targeted therapy medicines block the growth and spread of cancer because they interfere with processes in the cells that cause cancer to grow.

TIP

Targeted therapy causes less harsh or toxic side effects because it does not affect healthy rapidly dividing cells.

The most well-known targeted therapy is trastuzumab (marketed as Herceptin), a medicine that kills specific cancer cells that are HER2+ (HER2-positive). A protein called *human epidermal growth factor receptor 2* (HER2), which is found on the surface of the cancer cell, in large quantities can promote the rapid growth of cancer cells. Approximately 20–25 out of every 100 patients with breast cancer are HER2+ and are most likely to respond well to Herceptin treatment.

Figure 7-8 illustrates HER2 receptors.

It's difficult to predict how any one person will respond to a treatment. Therefore, targeted therapies were developed based on a particular group of factors that may be found on a tumor. Herceptin treatment was made possible through the results from clinical trials that show specific therapies to be more effective on certain types of breast cancer cells. Clinical trials have shown that Herceptin reduces the risk of HER2-positive breast cancers from coming back. In other words, individuals with HER2+ breast cancer get personalized treatment, which is as a result of *precision medicine* (see nearby sidebar for more on precision medicine).

Figure 7-9 illustrates how Herceptin works on HER2+ breast cancer cells.

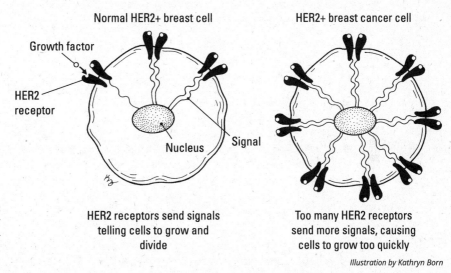

Normal HER2+ breast cell

Growth factor

HER2 receptor

Nucleus

Signal

HER2 receptors send signals telling cells to grow and divide

HER2+ breast cancer cell

Too many HER2 receptors send more signals, causing cells to grow too quickly

FIGURE 7-8: How cancer disrupts HER2+ breast cells.

Illustration by Kathryn Born

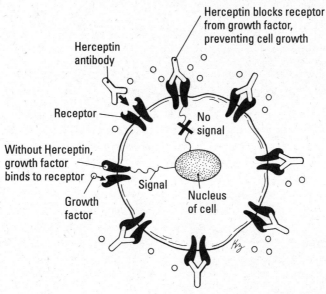

Herceptin blocks receptor from growth factor, preventing cell growth

Herceptin antibody

Receptor

No signal

Without Herceptin, growth factor binds to receptor

Signal

Growth factor

Nucleus of cell

FIGURE 7-9: Herceptin (antibody) action on HER2+ breast cancer.

Illustration by Kathryn Born

GLIMPSE OF THE FUTURE: PRECISION MEDICINE

Many people are diagnosed with a disease for which no proven treatment is available. There is much we do not know about diseases and how to find the best medicine to fight them. What is going on in our bodies or our cells that causes certain diseases to develop? Is there something in someone's DNA perhaps that makes a person especially vulnerable? Precision medicine focuses on finding the best medicine to treat a disease based on factors specific to a person:

- The person's genes

- Their lifestyle factors (non-genetic personal characteristics)

- Molecular (cell) characteristics of the disease

In 2015 President Barack Obama announced the Precision Medicine Initiative during his State of the Union address. This initiative has involved the recruitment of over 1 million individuals who volunteer their health information for researchers to develop specialized treatments for cancer on the basis of genetic and molecular profiles. This method of testing looks at each person's cancer tumor and studies the genetic characteristics as well as any unique proteins or biomarkers.

Precision medicine represents a "new model of scientific research" where patients are engaged in a partnership with researchers to find a cure for diseases that include cancer. The goal of precision medicine is to give the most effective treatment for each person's breast cancer that includes the following:

- Getting the best treatment results while avoiding unnecessary treatment and side effects.

- Developing therapies to target specific types of tumors and identify the individuals for which the treatment will be effective.

- Identifying contributing factors to help personalize the individual's breast cancer treatment. Factors that relate to the type of tumor will provide a better indication of prognosis and help tailor the treatment with the most benefit.

Researchers have learned over time that cancer develops as a result of genetic mutations in the cell, and this is due to a combination of environmental and genetic factors that cause cellular damage. That can lead to out-of-control cell growth, which leads to the development of tumors and sometimes the spread of those tumors to other parts of the body. The discovery of genetic mutations and the influence of environmental factors were the foundation for the birth of the science of precision medicine.

The idea of precision medicine is to put a stop to the "one-size-fits-all approach" to the design of medical treatments. In the future, medical treatments will be personalized according to differences in an individual's genes, lifestyles, and environments. The Food & Drug Administration (FDA) has already been approving medical treatments that are specific to patients' genetic profile of their cancer. Patients are receiving routine molecular testing — a collection of techniques used to analyze protein biological markers in the individual's genetic code and how their cells express their genes as proteins — by their oncology specialists to determine the best treatments to improve their survival and lower the risk of adverse reactions. The FDA will continue to oversee the accuracy of genetic tests using gene sequencing that includes *next-generation sequencing* (NGS).

Other targeted therapies besides Herceptin include the following:

>> **Bevacizumab (marketed as Avastin):** Used to treat colon cancer and ovarian cancer.

>> **Lapatinib:** Used to treat HER2+ metastatic breast cancer.

>> **Everolimus (marketed as Afinitor):** Used to treat kidney cancer, breast cancer, and brain cancer.

>> **Pertuzumab (marketed as Perjeta):** Used in combination with Herceptin and/or Taxotere to treat metastatic breast cancer.

>> **T-DM1 (marketed as Kadcyla):** Used to treat HER2+ metastatic breast cancer.

>> **Denosumab (marketed as Xgeva):** Used for treatment of secondary breast cancer in the bone.

Considering Clinical Trials

You may have completed a science project for a science fair in school to determine whether you could prove your *hypothesis* — an idea or explanation that you test through your study and experimentation. A *clinical trial* follows the same idea as your science project. It's a research project that tries to prove that a new treatment or medical procedure works in patients.

In pre-clinical trials, the medication or treatment is tested in a lab on cells or in animals. The success of pre-clinical trials determines whether the treatment is safe and will help people. Only then is a clinical trial initiated in patients. Before a clinical trial starts, it has to be approved, first by a group of independent scientists and then by a research ethics committee called the Institutional Review Board (IRB). These committees are often based at local hospitals and are made up of healthcare professionals and non-medical people. For breast cancer, different types of clinical trials look at different aspects of it, including the following:

» Ways to reduce the risk of getting breast cancer

» Diagnosing breast cancer

» Treating breast cancer

» Effects of a specific treatment on quality of life

» Complementary therapies (non-medical treatments), such as counseling, social support, diet, and physical activity

New medications go through several phases of testing on patients in clinical trials before they can be used as routine treatment for patients. You may be able to volunteer to take part in a clinical trial.

Randomized controlled trials (RCT)

A *randomized controlled trial* (RCT) is a type of trial where people who participate are randomly assigned to different groups given different treatments. Usually one group is given the standard cancer treatment (the treatment you would have even if you were not participating in a clinical trial). This group is also called the *control* group. The other group of participants receives the new treatment that is not standard treatment. This group is called the *experimental* group.

REMEMBER

Assignment to one group or the other is usually done by a computer in a process called *randomization*. Randomization prevents bias and assures the integrity of the experiment. If you decide to take part in an RCT clinical trial, neither you nor your doctor will be able to choose which type of treatment you will receive.

Placebos and double-blind trials

In a *double-blind trial*, a new medicine is compared with a *placebo* — a fake medicine that has no active ingredients but is made to look exactly like the medicine being tested.

When a placebo is used in a clinical trial it means that the effect of the new drug can be measured accurately through comparison. This is necessary because, strange as it may seem, some people may appear to feel better just because they are participating in a clinical trial. The reasons for this *placebo effect* are unknown, but some argue that improved symptoms occur because of frequent and close monitoring and optimism of patient and doctor.

If you decide to take part in a placebo/double-blind trial, neither you nor your doctor will know whether you are receiving the active treatment or placebo.

Length of clinical trials

Clinical trials can last less than a year or take place over several years. The length of a clinical trial depends on what they are looking at. At the end of the clinical trial, the results are made known, and that is when the results may support a new treatment into standard cancer care.

If you're randomly assigned to receive a new treatment during a clinical trial, there is a chance that the new treatment will help shrink or cure your cancer. But there is also a chance that the new treatment may have no effect on your cancer. There is also a chance that the new treatment could make you sick due to side effects, and still have no effect on your cancer. Because there is a chance of no effect of the new treatment, patients who have failed traditional treatment or are not eligible for traditional treatment are typically offered participation in clinical trials.

A bonus reason to take part in trials and experiments is that years from now, you may be able to say that you helped in the discovery and validation of a new treatment that could have significant benefit for future populations worldwide. Participating in clinical trials is really supporting the "greater good" of society.

Chapter 8

Breast Surgery

So, you're thinking about breast surgery — or perhaps surgery is already scheduled. Deciding on the best type of surgery can be overwhelming and can pose a dilemma. Here are a few questions to help you make a decision:

» Do you want to keep your breast or remove it (if applicable)?

» How will your breast look after a lumpectomy?

» How will your breast look after a mastectomy?

» Do you want breast reconstruction?

» Do you want breast reconstruction at the same time, or later?

» What type of breast reconstruction do you want? With or without implants?

» Do you want a tummy tuck so the tissue from your tummy can be used to form your breast?

» How much time can you take off from work?

» Who will support your family while you're recovering from surgery?

These questions are valid and their answers can have a huge impact on any decisions you make, regardless of what the surgeon may suggest.

Types of Breast Surgery

The most common types of breast surgery include the following:

» **Lumpectomy (partial mastectomy):** The tumor is removed from the breast along with a small border of healthy normal tissue.

» **Mastectomy (total or simple):** The entire breast is removed.

» **Modified radical mastectomy:** The entire breast and lymph nodes under the arm are removed.

» **Prophylactic mastectomy:** Occurs when a person chooses to remove one or both breasts because of familial or genetic risk factors.

» **Mastectomy with reconstruction:** This is where reconstruction is performed at the same time as removal of the breast. Many types of reconstruction include placement of a foreign material (implant or tissue expander) or use of your own tissue to reconstruct the breast.

Figure 8-1 illustrates how a tissue expander works.

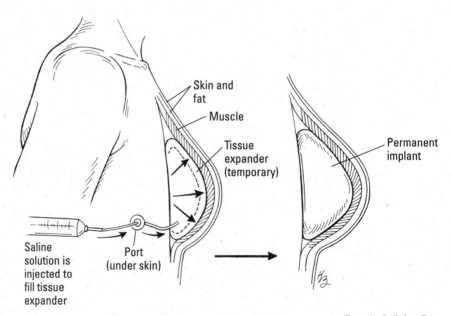

FIGURE 8-1: Tissue expander placed under skin and muscle and inflated with saline solution.

Saline solution is injected to fill tissue expander

Port (under skin)

Skin and fat

Muscle

Tissue expander (temporary)

Permanent implant

Illustration by Kathryn Born

>> **Sentinel lymph node biopsy:** The surgeon injects a blue and/or radioactive dye under the nipple area (the *subareolar* region) several hours prior to surgery. After injection, the breast is massaged for a few minutes to allow the dye to be taken up by the lymphatic system. The path of the dye will represent the drainage pattern of that breast.

During surgery the surgeon removes the tumor and, thanks to dyes, the surgeon is able to find whether any lymph nodes have picked up the dyes. The blue dye can be visualized with the eye, and the radioactive dye is tracked using an instrument called a *gamma probe.* The first lymph node to pick up both dyes is called the *sentinel* lymph node. The sentinel nodes are the first few lymph nodes into which a breast cancer or tumor drains. The blue dye gets from the breast tumor to the lymph nodes by way of the *lymph fluid* (blood plasma, proteins, glucose, and oxygen in the lymphatic vessels). The purpose of using the blue dye in sentinel lymph node biopsy is to identify the sentinel lymph nodes. Chapter 1 talks more about lymphatic vessels and lymph fluid.

The surgeon typically removes one to three nodes for testing. After your surgery, the pathologist will determine whether or not cancer has spread to those sentinel lymph nodes. This will help determine whether you will need more surgery to remove all the lymph nodes (a completion axillary lymph node dissection) and/or chemotherapy or radiation.

TIP

You may be worried about radiation exposure from the radioactive dye. Rest assured that the amount of dye and radiation is so small that it's safe to use in pregnant women that have breast cancer. It's equivalent to the amount of daily background radiation you get from the environment.

>> **Axillary lymph node dissection:** The surgeon removes most of the lymph nodes (levels one and two) from under the arm to determine how far the cancer cells have spread and to stop the spread. This procedure is done in large tumors or if there is known to be cancer in the lymph nodes (for example, after a positive result from a sentinel lymph node biopsy). Removing many of the lymph nodes under the arm increases your risk of having arm swelling, called *lymphedema.*

Preparing for Surgery

Regardless of which type of breast surgery you have, you will likely have questions for your surgeon. You should bring a list of your questions to your surgeon's visit to ensure that all concerns are discussed. Your surgeon will provide you with instructions on what things to avoid prior to surgery. It's important to understand the risks and how the procedure will be done.

The lumpectomy, mastectomy (total or radical modified), axillary dissection, and sentinel lymph node procedures generally don't require an *inpatient* stay, where you stay overnight at the hospital. These procedures are normally done as outpatient services, meaning the patient is not admitted to the hospital. That's right, you can probably go home the same day. However, individuals who are older or have multiple chronic diseases (called *comorbidity*) may be required to stay in the hospital for a night.

The lumpectomy procedure usually takes approximately one hour, with additional time needed for preparation and post-care. The total mastectomy procedure can take approximately an hour and a half, with additional preparation time and post-care. If you are having both breasts removed or having a mastectomy with tissue expander placement, the surgery time will be longer. Talk to your surgeon more about the time needed for your specific breast surgery. The preparations for axillary node dissection and sentinel lymph node biopsy are the same as those for a lumpectomy or mastectomy.

Talking to your surgeon before surgery

You will meet with your surgeon or team (usually consisting of an anesthesiologist, breast care nurse, or nurse navigator or coordinator) several days prior to your surgery (lumpectomy, mastectomy, axillary dissection). The team will talk to you about what will happen during the surgery. They will also lay out certain presurgical restrictions you need to follow. They may do this during your clinic appointment before surgery and again when you arrive at the hospital on the day of your surgery.

The surgeon will explain what they will do and what to expect when you recover from anesthesia. Don't forget to bring a list of questions to remind you of every concern you may have or information you would like to know. The more you know about what's going to happen, the less worry you will have. Understand the surgical procedure, risks, and side effects.

General surgery and anesthesia common risks and side effects include the following:

» Blood clots

» Heart attack

» Nausea and vomiting (usually occur immediately after surgery and may last for an additional day or two)

» Sore throat (during surgery a tube may be inserted into your throat to help you breathe, which may later cause a sore throat)

MARKING THE AREA WITH PEN

Your surgeon may use a marker pen to draw where the openings or incisions will be made on your breast the day of your surgery, just before you go to the operating room. This is helpful because you will know where they will cut, and the markings serve as a guide to know where to make the openings to remove the tumor or lymph nodes. The marks may be on the breast and/or under the arm.

Breast surgical risks and side effects include the following:

>> Bleeding

>> Hematoma (collection of blood under your skin)

>> Lymphedema (swelling in the arm on the same side of the breast cancer)

>> Negative reaction to anesthesia

>> Nerve pain

>> Numbness (sensory loss in upper arm and axilla)

>> Pain

>> Poor wound healing

>> Seroma (collection of fluid under your skin)

>> Shoulder stiffness

>> Swelling around the site of surgery

>> Wound infection

Pre-surgical restrictions

Anesthesia and surgery are delicate procedures, and they can be tricky. You must tell your surgeon about all medications (including herbal/natural supplements). These other substances can alter your body's metabolism of anesthetic agents, so your medical team needs to know whether to adjust the dose. Some medications can also interact with the anesthetic agents.

Here are some of the common risks of vitamins and nutritional supplements:

>> Vitamin E can slow blood clotting.

>> St. John's wort, Echinacea, ephedra, garlic, ginkgo, ginseng, kava, and valerian can all cause increased bleeding, affect blood glucose levels, and cause anesthesia.

Help your surgeon keep you safe during surgery by sharing the following information if it applies to you:

>> Any and all prescription medications, including patches and creams.

>> Any and all over-the-counter medications, herbs, vitamins, minerals, or natural or home remedies.

>> Whether you have allergies, including allergies to latex or adhesive tape.

>> Whether you have a pacemaker, automatic implantable cardioverter-defibrillator (AICD), or other heart device.

>> Whether you have sleep apnea.

>> Your willingness to receive a blood transfusion.

>> Whether you take a blood thinner such as aspirin, acetaminophen, ibuprofen, heparin, warfarin (Coumadin), clopidogrel (Plavix), and so on. Having thin blood can make surgery trickier. Make sure your surgeon knows *all* the medications you're taking.

>> Whether you take hormone replacement therapy (HRT).

>> Whether you have had a problem with anesthesia in the past.

>> Whether you smoke and how much and for how long.

>> Whether you drink alcohol and how much.

>> Whether you use recreational drugs, legal or otherwise.

Special Pre-Surgery Concerns

This section discusses some common pre-surgery concerns.

Alcohol consumption

You should abstain from drinking alcohol for at least 24 hours before surgery. Drinking a large amount of alcohol prior to surgery could affect you during surgery and your healing afterwards.

WARNING

If you are a heavy drinker of alcohol, it is important that you gradually start reducing the amount of alcohol you drink as soon as you know your surgery date. If you're an alcoholic and you stop drinking alcohol suddenly, you may experience withdrawal symptoms including delirium, seizure, and ultimately death. *Do not hide such information from your doctor.* If your surgeon is aware of the risk of you developing withdrawal symptoms, for example, medications can be prescribed to prevent them.

In addition, alcohol abuse also puts you at risk for bleeding, heart problems, infection, difficulty recovering post-surgery, being more dependent on nursing care, and potentially a longer hospital stay to manage complications.

It is crucial that you talk with your surgeon about your alcohol intake.

Smoking tobacco or cannabis

Your surgeon may ask you to stop smoking tobacco cigarettes prior to surgery. Smoking can lead to having problems with recovering from anesthesia and complications from slow healing. Nicotine starves the heart of oxygen by causing blood vessels to constrict, and, of course, oxygen-rich blood is needed not just for breathing but for healing.

The earlier you quit smoking before your surgery, the more you reduce your risk of smoking-related complications during and after surgery. It is best that you quit smoking at least 30 days prior to surgery or as long as possible prior to surgery. However, quitting a few days before surgery has been proven to still be somewhat beneficial. Even refraining from smoking as early as 12 hours prior to surgery improves heart and lung function and blood flow.

If you smoke cannabis (marijuana), you may want to argue that it's not cigarettes and you don't need to quit before surgery. However, cannabis has similar detrimental effects to nicotine during surgery. Smoking cannabis prior to surgery may cause the anesthesia to be more or less effective. It can also affect blood pressure in a similar way to nicotine because of increased carbon dioxide and reduced levels of oxygen in the blood.

This is another thing to not hide from your surgeon. Talk to your surgeon about tobacco or cannabis use.

Sleep apnea

If you are diagnosed with sleep apnea, then you must have completed a sleep study — a test used to diagnose sleep disorders. *Polysomnography* records your brain waves, the oxygen level in your blood, heart rate and breathing, as well as eye and leg movements during the study.

Sleep apnea is a common breathing disorder that may cause you to stop breathing for frequent short periods during your sleep. Obstructive sleep apnea (OSA) is the most common type. It occurs when the airway becomes completely blocked during sleep, causing no air or oxygen to come through to the nose or the mouth. What happens is the muscles in the back of your throat that support the soft palate, tonsils, tongue, and uvula (that piece of tissue hanging from the soft palate) become too relaxed. Relaxed muscles may cause the airway to close or narrow as you breathe in (inhale) and your oxygen intake may be inadequate for several seconds. That lowers the level of oxygen in the blood and causes carbon dioxide to build up in it.

Anesthesia also causes the muscles of the mouth and the throat to relax similar to the process that occurs in OSA. However, patients with OSA are more sensitive to the anesthesia dose than those who don't have OSA, and the muscles may become too relaxed. In some cases, patients with OSA may have difficulty recovering from the anesthesia.

WARNING

It is important to tell your surgeon if you have OSA to reduce your risk during surgery. Often your surgeon will have you meet with the anesthesiologist for you to be evaluated for the best type of anesthesia that will minimize surgery complications. If you're going to be admitted (inpatient surgery), you can most likely bring your own CPAP (continuous positive air way pressure) machine to the hospital to use.

Even if you don't have a diagnosis of OSA but suspect you have it, you should still let your surgeon know so you can be further evaluated. Common signs to report if you suspect that you have OSA include the following:

>> Excessive daytime sleepiness

>> Loud snoring

>> Observed pauses of breathing during sleep

>> Waking up suddenly choking, snorting, or gasping from sleep

>> Waking up with a dry mouth or sore throat

>> Insomnia or waking up during the night, restlessness, difficulty falling back to sleep

>> Morning headache

>> Forgetfulness and difficulty concentrating

>> Mood changes such as depression or irritability

>> High blood pressure

>> Nighttime sweating

>> Decreased libido

>> Going to the bathroom frequently during the night

Following a pre-surgery checklist

You will need a pre-operative exam (a *pre-op*) by your general practitioner (GP) or primary care provider (PCP) within 30 days from the date of your surgery. This exam is necessary to ensure that surgery can be performed, with safety being the priority. Your surgeon may request the following exam and tests from your GP or PCP:

>> Physical exam to check your general health

>> Blood tests to check your kidney and liver and evaluate your risk for increased bleeding during surgery

>> Chest X-ray to check the health of your lungs

>> Electrocardiogram (ECG) to check the health of your heart

As for what you can do on your own, here is a list of things to do to cut down on the risk of problems before surgery:

>> **Shave under your underarm:** If you are having lymph nodes removed under your arm, you may need to get rid of underarm hair on that side just before your surgery. Your nurse may give you hair removal cream or ask you to shave just before your surgery. Shaving the arms also reduces the risk of infection. Alternatively, you may be asked to clip the hair short and not actually shave it. Shaving may create small abrasions to the skin that can allow bacteria to enter. Some hospitals do the shaving during surgery, so ask at the pre-op assessment.

TIP

>> **Quit smoking and drinking:** Being diagnosed with breast cancer and confronted with surgery is a life-changing moment. Rather than see it as a stressful trigger for your worst habits, look at it as an opportunity to take stock of your lifestyle and as motivation to change behaviors. This time is a great opportunity for you to commit to quitting smoking and quitting or cutting back on alcohol to improve your quality of life for years to come. If you need help quitting smoking, call 1-800-Quit-Now. If you don't know how to quit smoking or drinking alcohol and need help, talk to your doctor about medical treatment options, such as being referred to community resources for assistance.

Be honest with your surgeon about how much alcohol you drink. Try to stop drinking once your surgery date is planned. Remember that you can gradually reduce your alcohol intake to avoid suddenly stopping.

WARNING

If you stop drinking alcohol and develop nausea, headache, increased anxiety, or difficulty sleeping, you must let your doctor know right away. These are signs of withdrawal that can be treated. Tell your doctor if you cannot stop drinking.

>> **Check your insurance:** Check with your health insurance company to make sure the surgical procedure is covered, whether you will have any out-of-pocket cost or deductible (and how much that will be), and whether there are any restrictions on where you should have the procedure done.

>> **Stop taking pain relievers:** Lay off the aspirin, naproxen (Aleve), ibuprofen (Advil), acetaminophen/paracetemol (Tylenol), and other blood-thinning medication at least one week prior to surgery to reduce risk of bleeding. There are exceptions for individuals who have had a recent stroke, heart attack, or a cardiac stent, where blood-thinning medications will be modified in preparation for surgery, but those decisions are directed by a *cardiologist* (specializing in the heart and blood vessels) or *hematologist* (specializing in blood and bone marrow).

>> **Stop eating and drinking:** Do not eat or drink after midnight on the day of the surgical procedure or eight hours before the surgical procedure to reduce the risk of food going into your lungs while under general anesthesia. It's important for you to check with your surgeon to determine the pre-op requirements.

>> **Bring a buddy:** Bring someone with you on the day of the surgical procedure. You will need someone to drive you home. Another pair of ears to listen to the postoperative and discharge instructions is also important, because you will still be under the effects of anesthesia when you're discharged. Anesthesia takes several hours to wear off.

During the Surgery

Both lumpectomy and mastectomy are usually performed using *general anesthesia,* the medicine–induced state of amnesia, analgesia, muscle paralysis, and sedation that will make you blissfully unaware of what's happening during the procedure and unable to feel any pain.

For a lumpectomy, the surgeon will make an opening over the tumor, or over the area that contains the wire from the needle localization (see Chapter 8), remove the tumor and surrounding healthy tissue, and send it to a pathologist for analysis. The surgeon will do a similar procedure for a sentinel lymph node biopsy or axillary dissection. The surgeon will close the openings on the breast or armpit with the intention to preserve the shape of the breast as much as possible using *sutures*, stitches that may dissolve on their own or need to be removed later by the surgeon.

If you're having a mastectomy, the surgeon will make a wider opening than necessary for a lumpectomy to remove the breast tissue. If you're getting breast reconstruction, they will remove the breast tissue and leave the skin of the breast, with or without the nipple depending on the type of reconstruction.

Post-Surgery Tips

After your surgery, you will wake up wearing an oxygen mask or nasal *cannula* (tubes into your nose) to give you extra oxygen. When you become fully awake, you will be taken to the recovery unit, where your blood pressure, pulse, and breathing will be monitored by a nurse.

REMEMBER

You may wake up quickly from anesthesia or you may feel groggy, dizzy, or sluggish for several hours after the surgery. That's why you really need to bring someone who can drive you home.

Drains and drips

When you wake up, you may have also *intravenous infusion* (IV), tubes going into you providing fluids, until you are eating and drinking again. And you may have one or more drains coming out from your mastectomy incision or under the arm from the axillary dissection. Drains help collect blood and fluid that collect at the surgery site. If this fluid is not released, it can cause swelling, bruising, and infection. Your surgeon may want you to empty your drain and measure the amount of fluid every day. It's important to write this information down on a piece of paper and bring it to your follow-up appointment. This will help determine when it's safe to remove the drain.

If you had a longer surgery, such as breast reconstruction, you may be given a *urinary catheter*, a tube into your bladder that collects urine. During your recovery, the nurse will remove the catheter prior to discharge or when you are able to move around on your own.

Going home

If you had a lumpectomy, sentinel lymph node biopsy, or simple mastectomy, you will be discharged to return home when your condition is *stable* — meaning that you have awakened; your blood pressure, pulse, and breathing are normal; and the dressing is secured with no signs of bleeding.

If you had an axillary lymph node dissection or mastectomy with reconstruction (tissue expander and implants), you may need to stay in the hospital for a day or two if you're experiencing pain or bleeding.

Expect to have the following when discharged:

>> A dressing (bandage) over the surgery site.

>> Some pain, numbness, and a pinching sensation in your underarm area.

>> Written instructions about post-surgical care, including caring for the incision and dressing and recognizing signs of infection.

>> Prescriptions for pain medication and possibly an antibiotic.

>> The incision or wound site may be sealed with Dermabond or another type of superglue for the skin. With wound glue, no wound care is needed except to clean the area with soap and water when instructed by your surgeon. Don't use ointments, creams, lotions, or powders over Dermabond glue. Don't scrub the glue or pick at it — it will fall off after a few weeks.

You may shower 48–72 hours after surgery, as instructed by the surgeon. The incisions can get soapy and wet, but avoid applying full showerhead pressure at the site. Have your back face the showerhead pressure. Wash the incision site gently with soap and water and pat dry. Don't submerge the surgical site in bathwater. If you have drains, ask your surgeon if you're allowed to shower or bathe with them in. Sometimes they want you to wait until the drains are removed (you can sponge bath in the meantime).

TIP

A surgical bra may be provided to provide improved support post-surgery. Keep wearing the surgical bra until your surgeon has instructed you to wear an alternative. It's important to avoid bras with underwire during recovery.

Restrictions on activity

For the first 48 hours, keep your arm movements to a minimum, especially if you had a sentinel lymph node biopsy or lymph node dissection. Your arms should not be used to support your body or lift anything heavy. After this, you may move your shoulder joint but only at shoulder level. Your doctor will further instruct you at your follow-up appointment about exercises that you should perform, or you may be referred to physical therapy.

You will have a follow-up appointment with your doctor, usually 7–14 days after surgery. Your surgeon will check the surgery site to ensure that it is healing well and discuss the pathology report or results from the surgery. Pathology results will help your surgeon to determine what treatments you need. Your doctor may recommend any of the following:

>> **More surgery:** It may be that the edges around your tumor still show microscopic evidence of cancer that could not be felt or seen with the naked eye (called *positive margin*).

>> **Medical oncologist:** This doctor can discuss other types of treatment, including endocrine therapy (if your cancer is estrogen- and/or progesterone receptor-positive), chemotherapy, or both. (See Chapters 10 and 11 for more.)

>> **Radiation oncologist:** This doctor can discuss radiation treatment to the breast or under the armpit. Radiation is usually recommended after lumpectomy or after a sentinel lymph node or axillary dissection pathology was positive for breast cancer cells. (See Chapter 9 for more.)

>> **Social worker:** You may want or need help finding resources to support your social and physical needs while receiving further treatment.

>> **Psychiatrist, counselor, or support group:** These can help you cope with the diagnosis and treatment of breast cancer.

TIP

A light diet is best for the first few days after surgery, as the medication used for general anesthesia can cause nausea. Begin by taking liquids slowly and progress to soups or Jell-O. You may start a regular diet when you feel ready.

REMEMBER

If you have pain or discomfort, take the medication given to you upon discharge and pay close attention to the instructions. Sometimes a narcotic will be prescribed, such as Tylenol with oxycodone (Percocet), hydrocodone (Vicodin), propoxyphene (Darvocet), or codeine (Tylenol #3) for pain control within the first five days after surgery. To prevent inflammation or swelling and to improve healing, your doctor may prescribe Ibuprofen, Aleve, or something else. Take pain medication with crackers, Jell-O, or after a meal. If you have no pain, don't take the medication. Alcohol and pain medication should not be taken together.

Chapter **9**

Radiation Therapy

There are several myths about radiation. One is that radiation exposure to the breast can be deadly. When properly done, it is not, so let's get that out of the way first of all. It's good to have a curious mind, but be skeptical too. Make sure there is evidence to back up every claim you hear before you believe it. It's an unfortunate human tendency to blame something to be the cause of disease or illness without all the facts to back it up. It is important to separate myth from reality.

Radiation therapy (or radiotherapy) is one type of treatment for breast cancer. For primary breast cancer — breast cancer that has not spread beyond the breast or lymph nodes under the arm — it uses controlled high-energy rays to destroy cancer cells that are in its path or that may be left behind in the breast or *axilla* (under armpit) after surgery. Many patients don't understand how or why tumor cells are left behind after surgery. They often come to clinic after and ask "why didn't you take it all out while you were in there?" Some tumors can be seen with the naked eye or felt with the hand, as they contain millions, sometimes billions of cancer cells. But many tumors can't be seen or felt, as they may only contain thousands of cells. This is why some microscopic sites of tumor can be left behind after surgery. Radiation is a great tool to help kill residual cells that can't be seen while sparing you from a large operation that would create a large physical defect.

Radiation is also used to treat secondary breast cancer, which is breast cancer that has spread beyond the breast and lymph nodes under the arm often into lung, liver, brain, and bone tissues. The goal of using radiation to treat secondary breast cancer is to control and slow down the spread of the cancer, relieve symptoms, and improve your quality of life.

According to National Comprehensive Cancer Network (NCCN) guidelines, the treatment of breast cancer with a lumpectomy must be followed by radiation treatment to reduce the risk of the cancer returning in the breast area. You may often hear this treatment called *adjuvant* radiation or *additional* therapy. Adjuvant therapy can be chemotherapy or radiation therapy given *after* surgery. *Neoadjuvant therapy* (given before surgery) and *adjuvant therapy* (given after surgery) are common terms in cancer treatment.

There are exceptions to this rule. Your doctor may not recommend radiation because the risk outweighs the benefits for the following reasons:

>> You previously had radiation to that breast (there is a lifetime amount of radiation you can receive to maintain safe limits).

>> You are pregnant.

>> You are 70 years or older (your breast cancer is unlikely to recur in your remaining lifetime and so radiation will offer no therapeutic benefit).

>> You have multiple chronic illnesses.

REMEMBER

You may be offered radiation therapy based on your situation. Your *radiation oncologist* (a radiation cancer specialist) will consider the stage, grade, and size of your cancer, as well as your age and whether you have any other chronic diseases before making a recommendation for radiation.

How Radiation Therapy Works

Radiation treats the site where the breast cancer started with high-energy rays produced by a machine called a *linear accelerator* or LINAC. The linear accelerator focuses the high-energy rays onto the chest wall in the area where the tumor is (or was, if you've had surgery) to kill cancer cells while sparing most of the surrounding healthy normal tissue. It has built-in safety measures to ensure that it doesn't deliver a higher dose of rays than prescribed and is routinely checked by a medical physicist to ensure it's working properly.

Even though the linear accelerator is given in such a way as to have the greatest effect on cancer cells, it can also cause injury to healthy normal tissue — which is generally able to recover and repair itself. Radiation therapy is a highly specialized treatment and may not be available in every hospital or community. You should receive treatment at the closest radiation center where you will be treated as an outpatient.

Radiation therapy is usually given after a lumpectomy if you are not receiving chemotherapy. If you *are* receiving chemotherapy, you have to wait till the treatment has ended before you can start radiation. There is usually a 30-day delay before the start of radiation treatment, after surgery or chemotherapy. However, some people may have to wait longer depending on how fast their wounds after surgery are taking to heal, or for other medical reasons.

You'll first see the radiation oncologist in the outpatient department to talk about your treatment. Once the treatment, its benefits, risks, and potential side effects have been fully explained to you, you'll be asked to sign a consent form. A further appointment is then made to plan your treatment.

Radiation therapy is done at a radiation treatment center or hospital. To reduce risk, radiation treatment is actually divided into several courses of small treatments — getting the total dose of radiation at one time would cause harm to the body. Therefore, the treatment is split into equal small doses, called *fractions*, usually delivered every weekday over three to six weeks (with a rest on the weekend), depending on your treatment plan. The fraction given is usually the same each time.

Radiation therapy for primary breast cancer can be given in different ways and in different doses, depending on your treatment plan. The ultimate goal of radiation is to provide local or regional control of the breast cancer. Failure to achieve tumor control can result in the likelihood of breast cancer spreading to other parts of the body, severe physical limitation, or even death.

The main types of radiation are as follows:

>> **External beam radiotherapy:** This is the most common type of radiation therapy given to treat primary breast cancer. The high-energy rays are delivered from the linear accelerator with the beam directed to the body through the skin of the breast or under the armpit. The radiation treatment is focused on the area where the tumor was or is and some normal surrounding tissue will be radiated.

>> **Intensity modulated radiotherapy (IMRT):** Radiation intensity can be modified with IMRT during treatment in order to protect healthy normal tissue around the cancer in comparison to conventional radiation therapy such as external beam radiation. Because of the flexibility IMRT provides, higher doses of radiation can be given to the tumor site. IMRT is also called *conformal* radiation because it changes the shape of the beam to mirror the

tumor. Conventional or external beam radiation therapy delivers high-energy rays with uniform intensity across the area of your cancer, increasing the risk of healthy normal tissue injury. IMRT is able to more precisely delivery radiation than external beam.

>> **Radiation therapy boost:** This is a technique of giving the patient one or more extra radiation treatments after the regular sessions of radiation treatment are completed. Radiation boost has been very effective in keeping breast cancer from coming back. If you're having IMRT, the boost will be included in the planning strategy of the radiation to be delivered at a higher dose in the area when your whole breast is being treated. For conventional radiation, the boost will be given at the end of radiation sessions and will typically be five to eight extra sessions. Radiation boost is typically offered to patients in their forties or younger because research shows that they have the most to benefit. However, all ages of patients can have a lower risk of breast cancer coming back when they receive the radiation boost.

Other types of radiation therapy are less commonly used and may not be widely available:

>> **Respiratory gating:** This involves taking a deep breath at a specific time in your breathing cycle and holding the breath for a period of time at each session of external beam radiation. The goal of respiratory gating is to protect the heart and chest wall if the radiation site is to the left side or left breast. The breath-holding technique helps protect healthy tissues under the breast, which can reduce long-term side effects for the heart, such as heart disease.

>> **Brachytherapy:** The radiation source is placed inside the body at the site to be treated, therefore protecting the skin from radiation burns. Hollow narrow tubes or a small balloon are placed where the breast tissue has been removed. Then radioactive wires are inserted in the tubes or into the balloon and left for a short time each day or for a few days. You may be treated as an inpatient, depending on the type of brachytherapy you have, due to active radiation exposure.

>> **Intraoperative radiation:** Another way of giving internal radiation as seen with brachytherapy. This type of treatment uses low-energy rays from the machine in the operating room during a lumpectomy or breast conserving surgery. The radiation is given directly to the site where the cancer was removed. Only one dose of radiation is given per treatment. Sometimes you may receive this dose as the only radiation you will get; other times continuing with external beam radiation for a short duration is necessary. This type of radiation is not commonly used or available.

Planning for Radiation Treatment

Your treatment planning team will determine the treatment area for the radiation. The timing and amount of radiation will depend on your individual situation. Normally, radiation therapy is offered in three treatment options:

>> After a lumpectomy or breast conserving surgery.

>> After a mastectomy. Radiation is given to the chest wall and underarm area because the tumor was large, the tumor was close to the chest wall and cancer cells may still be present, or because cancer cells were found in the lymph nodes under the arm and surrounding areas.

>> Radiotherapy to the lymph nodes will be done if cancer is found in the lymph nodes under the arm or above the collarbone.

A radiation treatment planning team usually consists of the following:

>> **Radiation physicist:** A radiation physicist is a specialist who uses applied physics techniques in the use of radiation in the diagnosing and treatment of disease and ensuring safety.

>> **Dosimetrist:** A dosimetrist specializes in radiation treatment machines and equipment, and has the education and expertise in generating radiation dose distributions and dose calculations in collaboration with the medical physicist and radiation oncologist.

>> **Radiation oncologist:** A radiation oncologist is a doctor who specializes in radiation therapies for cancer patients.

Your radiotherapy team calculates how much radiation is needed to treat your breast cancer. A planning mammogram or CT scan may be used to show the breast tumor and the structures around it. Before treatment begins, the radiotherapy team carefully plans your external beam radiotherapy (most commonly used technique). This means working out how much radiation you need to treat the cancer and exactly where you need it.

After planning your radiation treatment, the treatment team may put ink marks on your skin to make sure they treat the same area every day. Sometimes pinpoint-sized tattoo marks are used for markings. Your treatment team may further outline areas on your breast or armpit to limit radiation doses or to avoid completely. This process is called *contouring*. The team finalizes the plan for the radiation using advanced computer software.

As always, you should know as much as you can about your treatment. Ask your doctor about radiation therapy for your breast cancer. Some of the questions you can ask include the following:

>> Why are you recommending radiation therapy for me?

>> What will the treatment involve and how long will I have to be treated?

>> Which areas will be treated?

>> Will the radiation therapy change the shape and texture of my breast?

>> Are there any other treatment options?

>> What are short-term or long-term side effects from the radiation?

>> What can I use to soothe my skin?

>> Will I need to take time off work during the radiation treatments?

>> Can I get transportation help to and from the radiation center or hospital?

>> Will having radiation to my breast affect my chances of having breast reconstruction later?

>> Whom can I contact for emotional support?

>> Is there a number I can call to speak to someone on your team anytime I experience new symptoms or have concerns?

Things to Do before Radiation Therapy

Here is a list of items you should check off before you enter on a course of radiation therapy:

>> Tell your oncologist about any and all medications, herbs, vitamins, and supplements that you're taking, to ensure that these substances don't cause a complication during treatment.

>> Go ahead and schedule your appointments for your radiation sessions when your treatment plan is given to you. This will ensure that you get the times that are convenient, especially if you have a work schedule.

>> It's best to schedule your appointments at the same time every day so you can get into a routine, and your body will get accustomed to internal changes as well.

>> Keep all your appointments. If you discover that you may have difficulty getting to your appointment due to lack of transportation, severe illness, or a pre-planned vacation, inform your oncologist.

Some radiation centers do offer assistance with transportation to and from treatment. Talk to your oncology nurse or oncologist if you anticipate transportation difficulties.

TIP

Post-Radiation Skincare

You must practice good skincare during and after radiation at the area being treated. Your skin may become temporarily burned during your treatment, but this almost always heals over time. Your radiation oncology team will provide you with special instructions for skincare, which you must follow to reduce the risk of severe skin reactions. The special instructions for skincare will be customized for you, but may include the following:

>> Wash the area treated gently with warm water using a mild soap and pat the skin dry with a soft towel.

>> Have a shower instead of a bath.

>> Have the shower run onto your back rather than your front.

>> Use a non-perfumed deodorant.

>> Use mild and gentle moisturizers to keep the skin soft. If you're not sure what to use, ask your oncologist.

>> Avoid exposing the treated area treated to extreme temperature such as ice packs, heating pads, saunas, and so on.

>> Avoid exposing the treated area to sun while receiving radiation treatment and afterwards, to reduce risk of skin reactions.

>> Avoid sunburn to the area being treated by using a sunscreen with SPF of 50 or higher. Apply the sunscreen even if you'll have clothes over the area because the sun's rays can penetrate clothing.

>> Avoid swimming during and shortly after treatment until any skin reactions have healed. Chemicals in the swimming pool can irritate the skin and cause a skin reaction. If you swim regularly and will have difficulty abstaining from swimming, talk to your oncologist.

>> Wear a soft cotton bra or vest to avoid friction or rubbing of the skin, which can worsen skin reaction. If you had a total mastectomy and are wearing a silicone prosthesis, it may be more comfortable to switch it to a lightweight prosthesis.

REMEMBER

If you develop a skin reaction, it should heal within three to four weeks of your last treatment. If it doesn't heal within this time, or if you have a more severe reaction such as skin peeling or blistering, contact your radiotherapy team, breast care nurse, primary care provider, or general practitioner for advice.

Radiation Therapy Side Effects

The side effects of radiation may be different for everyone, with some more common than others. Most of the side effects are immediate and temporary (called *immediate*), but some may be permanent or may linger for many months or years after receiving treatment (called *late*).

Immediate side effects can occur during treatment or up to six months after treatment has completed. The following sections cover these side effects.

Skin reactions

You may notice redness on the skin like a sunburn, itching, tenderness, and darkening of the skin at the treatment site. These changes usually occur within 10–14 days after starting treatment, but may happen near the end or when you receive the radiation boost. You may gradually notice peeling and flaking of the skin, and this may later develop into a blister, with a weepy skin reaction, but many people don't experience such severe skin reactions.

The level of skin reaction to radiation depends on the following:

>> The strength of the dose of radiation received

>> Skin type

>> Existing skin conditions such as eczema or psoriasis

REMEMBER

You must tell your radiation oncologist if you have any specific skin conditions to help reduce your risk of severe skin reactions.

Change in breast size and consistency

The breast may appear to be firmer, harder, or even thicker after radiation. Some women even notice that the radiated breast appears higher or to be lifted after radiation therapy and doesn't match the other breast.

Swelling or edema of the breast

Swelling may occur during treatment, in which you may feel your chest swollen or your breast feels uncomfortable. Sometimes the swelling settles after a few weeks, but if it continues, talk to your oncologist about it. Sometimes the oncologist may want you to be assessed by a *lymphedema therapist*, who performs manual lymphatic drainage using special massage techniques to move fluid into working lymph nodes, where they are drained.

Pain in the breast area

This kind of pain may feel like sharp twinges or aches in the breast/chest area or under the armpit. Such pains are usually mild and may continue after radiation has completed, but the frequency of the pain will gradually reduce over time. You may experience shoulder pain/discomfort or stiffness if you had radiation under the armpit.

The Importance of Exercising

REMEMBER

It's important to do arm and shoulder exercises during and several weeks after your radiation therapy to reduce stiffness or discomfort. These exercises are usually provided by your breast surgeon or radiation oncologist. See Chapter 18 for more information on exercises. This section suggests some exercises that can help after breast radiation or breast surgery.

Warm-up and cool down exercises

» **Shoulder shrugs:** Shrug your shoulders up towards your ears and lower them downward gently. Keep your arms loose or relaxed at your side while doing this exercise.

» **Shoulder circling:** Shrug your shoulders up towards your ears, then circle them back and forward then down toward the sides. If you have tightness across your chest or at the incision site, use smaller circles, but increase to larger circles as the tightness decreases. You may find that circling backward may cause your chest to feel tighter across your chest than the forward direction. Keep doing the exercises and you will have less chest tightness in both directions.

Basic exercises to do in the first week after surgery or radiation and beyond

» **Bent arm:** Raise both your arms forward so they are at right angles to your body. Bend your elbows and rest your hands lightly on your shoulders. Lower your elbows slowly, then raise them again. Alternative: Rest your hands on your shoulders but take your elbows out to the sides. Lower your elbows slowly, then raise them again.

» **Back scratching:** Hold your arms out to your sides and bend your arms from the elbow. Slowly reach up behind your back to just under your shoulder blades.

» **Hands behind the head (winging it):** Place your hands behind your head with elbows together in front of your face. Bring your elbows back so they're pointing out to the sides, then return to the beginning position.

Advanced exercises for the second week after surgery or radiation and beyond

» **W-exercise:** Form a *W* with your arms out to your side with palms facing forward. Bring your hands up to make them even to your face. Raise your arms to the most comfortable position. Bring your shoulder blades together (pinch) then downward, as if you are squeezing a pen between your shoulder blades.

» **Wall climbing:** Stand close to the wall with your feet apart, facing the wall. Put both hands on the wall at shoulder level. Looking straight ahead, gradually walk your fingers up the wall as far as you can, feeling a stretch but not pain. Hold and count to ten. Slide your fingers back to shoulder level before repeating the exercise. Try to get higher each time.

» **Side wall crawls:** Stand sideways with your affected side nearest the wall. Put your hand on the wall, keeping your elbow bent and your shoulders relaxed. Looking straight ahead, gradually walk your fingers up the wall as far as you can, allowing your elbow to straighten. Hold there and count to ten, then lower your hand back down.

» **Arm lifts:** Lie on the bed or floor with a cushion or pillow to support your head. While lying down, take three or four really deep breaths and concentrate on relaxing your shoulders so they are not hunched up towards your ears. Clasp your hands together or hold onto a stick or broom handle. Keeping your elbows straight, lift your arms up and over your head as far as you feel comfortable. Hold them there and count to ten, then lower your arms slowly. Alternative: If you have difficulty lying down — for example, because of breathlessness — you can do this exercise in a sitting position, leaning back in your chair.

>> **Elbow push:** Lie on your back with your hands behind your head and elbows out to the sides. Gently push your elbows downwards into the bed or floor as far as is comfortable. Hold and count to ten, then relax. This exercise is particularly helpful if you go on to have radiotherapy because the treatment will often require you to be in a similar position.

TIP

Do ten repetitions of each exercise five times a day until you regain full range of motion of your shoulder and arms.

Tiredness and fatigue

Generally, radiation to the breast is well tolerated, and many can in fact go to work while receiving radiation. However, having to go to radiation five days per week can be tiring when you add it to your job and home schedule, and may be physically overwhelming. In addition to the usual tiredness, radiation itself can cause *fatigue* — extreme tiredness and exhaustion that doesn't go away with sleep or rest. Fatigue can affect you emotionally and physically and may add to the fatigue you may already have from surgery or chemotherapy. Fatigue may occur during or after radiation.

REMEMBER

Everyone is different, and the level of fatigue and recovery can also be different. Know your limits and don't expect too much of yourself.

Lymphedema

This is swelling in the breast area as described earlier, but in this case it's also in the arm and hand, caused by the accumulation of lymph fluid in the surface tissues of the body. Lymphedema can occur post-surgery and during and after radiation. If you experience symptoms of tightness, fullness, or heaviness in these areas, talk to your oncologist right away. Lymphedema can occur for the long term, but you can control it with manipulation strategies and appropriate treatment. However, it may not completely go away.

Change in breast shape, size, and color

Usually when you have radiation after a lumpectomy, the breast tissue on the side of the breast that was treated will feel firmer, or the breast may shrink or appear to be "perkier" or lifted. This occurs because the breast has a rounded shape, and it's not possible to distribute perfectly even doses of radiation over the whole area.

The change in your breast shape is normal — don't worry. But if you're concerned with differences in the size of your breast, talk to your surgeon.

Hair loss in the armpit or chest area

Radiation therapy under the armpit will cause your hair under your arm to fall out, and for men it will cause chest hair to fall out. The hair under the arm and chest often regrows, but not always.

Sore throat

If you had radiation treatment near your collarbone you may experience sore throat or have difficulty swallowing during or after treatment. If this happens, talk to your radiation oncologist. Sometimes you may even have to take pain medicine (liquid form preferred) before eating to minimize throat discomfort.

Late side effects

The preceding sections discussed immediate side effects. Here we'll look at side effects that may develop several months or years after radiation treatment. Improved techniques such as IMRT and accuracy in marking the location that will be treated help minimize late side effects.

Dry cough

If part of your lung is radiated, it may cause a "radiation cough" — a dry cough that can often develop and last for several years after radiation has ended.

Fibrosis under the arm

Fibrosis under the arm is caused by radiation hardening the tissue under the arm, causing accumulation of scarring. When fibrosis is severe, the breast can appear noticeably smaller and firmer, and this can happen several months after completing radiation. Sometimes tiny broken blood vessels can be seen under the skin, called *telangiectasia*, which is currently untreatable.

Tenderness over the ribs during treatment

This can occur during and after treatment but may gradually improve over time. Radiation can cause pain that feels like arthritis-like inflammation to develop around the area that connects the sternum to the ribs. Sometimes tenderness over the ribs can feel like chest pain. If you feel tenderness or chest pain, inform your radiation oncologist.

Fibrosis of the upper lung

Fibrosis (scarring) may develop in the lung in rare cases.

Heart problems

WARNING

Although special precautions are taken to protect the tissues of the heart during radiation, there is a risk of developing heart problems in the future. Heart problems can be due to scarring/fibrosis of the heart muscle that was radiated. The scarred portion of the heart will not work as well, and this can lead to heart failure or heart attacks. Some of the major heart problems that can occur include heart attack from clogged blood vessels or even death due to reduced blood supply to the heart, called *ischemia*. The higher the radiation dose, the higher the risk of heart problems.

Weakening of bones

Bones in the area of the radiation treatment, such as collarbone or rib fractures, may weaken and fracture.

Tingling, numbness, and pain in the arm

These side effects are caused by nerve injury and can result in some loss of movement.

Chapter 10

Chemotherapy

Chemotherapy refers to using anti-cancer (*cytotoxic*) drugs to destroy cancer cells. The drugs circulate in the bloodstream around the body and work by disrupting the growth of cancer cells.

Chemotherapy can work wonders, but it often gets bad press from friends, family, and acquaintances for its side effects. And true, it has some. So do many medications. Tylenol or acetaminophen (used for pain) can cause nausea, rash, and a headache. Metformin (used for treating diabetes) can cause diarrhea, headache, nausea/vomiting, and a rash. And a medicine like docetaxel (chemotherapy medicine used for breast cancer) can cause diarrhea, nausea/vomiting, fatigue, and nail changes. Chemotherapy works by killing off cancer cells, but unfortunately certain normal cells in your body are also damaged by chemotherapy, which is what causes the side effects. Scientists, doctors, and the Food and Drug Administration (FDA) work hard to study chemotherapeutic agents to make sure the benefits outweigh the risks to people before approving them for use.

Different Types of Chemotherapy and How They Work

Chemotherapy comes in three main categories:

>> **Neoadjuvant chemotherapy:** This is chemotherapy that is given prior to surgery to shrink a tumor to a smaller size. Operating on a smaller tumor may make surgery more feasible or less disfiguring. It's also given to determine how sensitive the tumor is to that type of chemotherapy. The goal of this type of chemotherapy is to work toward a cure, often in combination with other treatments.

>> **Adjuvant chemotherapy:** This type is given after surgery to reduce the chance of the cancer spreading or coming back. It destroys any cancer cells that may be in the body. This type of chemotherapy may also be given for breast tumors that have come back. As with neoadjuvant chemotherapy, the goal of this type of chemotherapy is to work toward a cure.

>> **Palliative chemotherapy:** This kind is given when the breast cancer has spread to other organs or has progressed to stage IV. It may be given indefinitely in order to prolong life or suppress or control the tumor and reduce symptoms. The goal of this type of chemotherapy is for comfort—to relieve pain that may be caused by the tumor invading organs of the body, but *rarely to cure.*

Common chemotherapy medications used for adjuvant and neoadjuvant chemo-therapy (often used in combinations of two or three together) include the following:

>> Carboplatin (Paraplatin)

>> Cyclophosphamide (Cytoxan)

>> Docetaxel (Taxotere)

>> Doxorubicin (Adriamycin)

>> Epirubicin (Ellence)

>> 5-fluorouracil (5-FU)

>> Paclitaxel (Taxol)

Common chemotherapy used for advanced breast cancer or for palliation or com-fort care (often used for treating breast cancer that has spread to other parts of the body) include the following:

>> Albumin-bound paclitaxel (nab-paclitaxel or Abraxane)

>> Capecitabine (Xeloda)

>> Carboplatin (Paraplatin)

>> Cisplatin (Platinol)

>> Docetaxel (Taxotere)

>> Eribulin (Halaven)

>> Gemcitabine (Gemzar)

>> Ixabepilone (Ixempra)

>> Liposomal doxorubicin (Doxil)

>> Mitoxantrone (Novantrone)

>> Paclitaxel (Taxol)

>> Vinorelbine (Navelbine)

As you can see already, many (and we mean *many*) types of chemotherapy medications are used for treating breast cancer.

But how do they work? To understand that, it helps to look at the cell cycle. Chemotherapy, after all, acts on the cells.

The cells in your body reproduce by cell division, meaning one cell divides into two identical cells. Almost every time they do so, the two new cells are identical to the parent cell. But, as mentioned in Chapter 1, sometimes there can be damage to the instructions that tell the cell what to do, leading to the new cells being different in some way to the parent cell. Such a change is called a *mutation*. A mutation can cause what had been a normal cell to evolve into a tumor that is malignant or cancerous.

As you may (or may not) recall from biology class, there are five phases in the cell cycle:

1. **G1 Phase, regular life:** This is when cells increase in size, produce RNA, and synthesize protein. This phase is also called the *G1 checkpoint* because it ensures that all cell activity is ready for DNA replication.

2. **S Phase, DNA replication:** This is when two similar daughter cells are produced and each contains the complete DNA instructions for replication.

3. **G2 Phase:** Growth of the cell in preparation for division — the cell continues to grow and produce new proteins. This phase is also called the *G2 checkpoint* because it determines whether the cell can proceed to enter M Phase and divide.

4. **M Phase, mitosis and cytokines:** *Mitosis* is the process that duplicates the genome in a cell and separates it into identical halves. *Cytokinesis* is the process where the cell's *cytoplasm* — the fluid that fills a cell and serves several functions that are key to cellular health and productivity — divides to form two *daughter* cells (as discussed in Chapter 1).

5. **G0 Phase, cell cycle rest:** This is when a cell will leave the cycle and quit dividing. It can be a temporary resting period or a more permanent one.

REMEMBER

A breast cancer cell is a damaged (mutated) cell that continues to duplicate in an uncontrolled manner, forming a tumor that can get larger and eventually spread to other parts of the body. Because chemotherapy works by attacking different cell cycle phases, the most effective chemotherapies for breast cancer must be able to work at every cycle of the cell (except G0, the rest cycle).

Table 10-1 shows the different classes of chemotherapy medications used to treat breast cancer:

>> *Anthracycline* antibiotics are a type of antibiotic that comes from certain types of *Streptomyces* bacteria. Anthracyclines are used to treat many types of cancer. Anthracyclines damage the DNA in cancer cells, causing them to die. Daunorubicin, doxorubicin, and epirubicin are anthracyclines.

>> *Taxanes* are a type of drug that blocks cell growth by stopping mitosis (cell division). Taxanes interfere with *microtubules* (cellular structures that help move chromosomes during mitosis). They are used to treat cancer. A taxane is a type of mitotic inhibitor and a type of antimicrotubule agent.

>> *Antimetabolites* are a type of drug that is very similar to natural chemicals in a normal biochemical reaction in cells but different enough to interfere with the normal division and functions of cells.

>> *Alkalating agents* cause replacement of hydrogen by an alkyl group to inhibit cell division and growth.

>> *Antineoplastics* inhibit or prevent the growth and spread of tumors or malignant cells.

>> *Vinka alkaloids* are a type of drug that blocks cell growth by stopping mitosis (cell division). Vinca alkaloids interfere with microtubules (cellular structures that help move chromosomes during mitosis). A vinca alkaloid is a type of mitotic inhibitor and a type of antimicrotubule agent.

>> *Epothilones* are obtained from bacteria and interfere with cell division.

TABLE 10-1   ## Chemotherapy Medications and What They Target

Class	S Phase	M Phase	G1 Phase	G2 Phase
Anthracycline antibiotics	Doxorubicin (Adiamycin)	Doxorubicin (Adiamycin)	Doxorubicin (Adiamycin)	Doxorubicin (Adiamycin)
	Epirubicin (Ellence)	Epirubicin (Ellence)	Epirubicin (Ellence)	Epirubicin (Ellence)
	Liposomal doxorubicin (Doxil)			
Taxanes		Paclitaxel (Taxol)		Paclitaxel (Taxol)
		Docetaxel (Taxotere)		Albumin-bound paclitaxel (nab-paclitaxel or Abraxane)
		Albumin-bound paclitaxel (nab-paclitaxel or Abraxane)		
Antimetabolites	Methotrexate (Trexall)			
	5-fluorouracil (5-FU)			
	Gemcitabine (Gemzar)			
	Capecitabine (Xeloda)			
Alkalating agents	Cyclophosphamide (Cytoxan)	Cyclophosphamide (Cytoxan)	Cyclophosphamide (Cytoxan)	Cyclophosphamide (Cytoxan)
	Mitomycin (Mitomycin C)	Mitomycin (Mitomycin C)	Mitomycin (Mitomycin C)	Mitomycin (Mitomycin C)
	Cisplatin (Platinol)	Cisplatin (Platinol)	Cisplatin (Platinol)	Cisplatin (Platinol)
	Carboplatin (Paraplatin)	Carboplatin (Paraplatin)	Carboplatin (Paraplatin)	Carboplatin (Paraplatin)
Antineoplastics		Eribulin (Halaven)		Mitoxantrone (Novantrone)
				Eribulin (Halaven)
Vinka alkaloids		Vinorelbine (Navelbine)		
Epothilones		Ixabepilone (Ixempra)		Ixabepilone (Ixempra)

THE "RED DEVIL" CHEMO

You may have heard your oncologist say that you will get a *red devil* combination therapy. Don't you dare take that statement literally! The red devil is Adriamycin. Adriamycin treatment got that nickname because the solution is red in color and can have many undesirable side effects, including low red blood cells (anemia), low white blood cells (neutropenia), low platelets, mouth sores, hair loss, changes to fingernails and toenails, and discolored urine.

REMEMBER

Unfortunately, chemotherapy medications can't tell the difference between a normal cell and a cancer cell. They kill actively growing and dividing cells. Cancer cells actively grow and divide more often than normal cells, so they are more likely to be killed by chemotherapy. And even though normal cells do sometimes die, they are much better at repairing damage caused by chemotherapy than cancer cells.

How Chemotherapy Is Given

Chemotherapy is typically given *intravenously*, or in the vein, as an infusion over several hours or as an injection over a few minutes. Some are given weekly.

It's usually given in *cycles*. Each cycle of treatment is followed by a rest period to give your body (your normal cells) time to recover before the next cycle. Your treatment team will draw your blood just before starting the next cycle to make sure your blood cell counts are normal.

Some cycles of chemotherapy may be given weekly, every two weeks, or every three weeks, and in combination. The order that the chemotherapy is administered may differ based on your treatment plan. Often the cycles are shortened, with minimum rest periods, because research has shown that *dose-dense chemotherapy* can reduce the chance of cancer coming back.

Adjuvant and neoadjuvant chemotherapies are usually administered over a period of three to six months, depending on whether the medication is proving effective or not. For patients with advanced or stage IV breast cancer, chemotherapy is given continuously but may be changed or stopped depending on how it's working or if the patient is tolerating the side effects.

Common Side Effects of Different Chemotherapies

The side effects you may experience from chemotherapy depend on the type of medications used. As mentioned, chemotherapy kills actively dividing normal cells. Most cells in the body divide and multiply over time, but the ones that turn over quickly are affected most by chemotherapy. These include the skin, hair, nails, mouth, lining of stomach and digestive system, and bone marrow (which makes new blood cells). So, many of the most common side effects occur in these organs, plus others.

Some chemotherapies may cause one effect, and others won't. For example, paclitaxel can cause injury to the nerves, brain, and spinal cord that can lead to *peripheral neuropathy*, a nerve problem that causes pain, numbness, tingling, swelling, or muscle weakness in different parts of the body. Doxorubicin can cause heart damage, including *cardiomyopathy*, chronic disease of the heart muscle. Just because a chemotherapy has a listed side effect doesn't mean it will definitely occur. But it is important to be aware of the common side effects so that you can report the signs or symptoms as early as possible to your doctor. Your doctor may adjust your dose, skip a dose, or change the therapy altogether if needed.

Table 10-2 lists chemotherapy side effects as they relate to the body system.

TABLE 10-2   **Common Side Effects of Chemotherapy Based on Body System**

Body System	Side Effects
Bone marrow	Tiredness or fatigue
	Bruising
	Bleeding
	At risk for infections: Signs and symptoms include high temperature or lower than normal temperature, feeling cold or chilly, cough, aching muscles, sore throat, pain when passing urine
Digestive system	Mouth sores
	Taste changes
	Diarrhea
	Constipation
	Poor appetite
	Weight loss

(continued)

TABLE 10-2 *(continued)*

Body System	Side Effects
Hair, skin, and nails	Hair is thinner
	Hair loss on head and body, including eyebrows
	Dry skin
	Sensitive skin
	Skin rash
	Nail ridges
	Brittle nails
	Nails with white lines
Central and peripheral nervous system	Numbness or pain in hands and feet
	Hearing loss, especially high-pitched sounds
	Ear ringing
Kidneys	Renal failure (kidneys not working properly)
	Edema (swelling or abnormal accumulation of fluid) can occur all over the body. People will be more "puffy" than usual in face/hands/legs. Patients often notice it in their legs the most, as gravity settles the most fluid here.
Liver	Liver failure
	Jaundice (yellow discoloration of skin)
	Bleeding easily
	Swollen abdomen
	Confusion or disorientation
	Sleepiness
Heart	Irregular heartbeat
	Fast heartbeat (tachycardia)
	Shortness of breath
	Dry cough
	Fatigue
	Swelling of hands and feet (edema)
	Congestive heart failure (heart is not pumping sufficient blood)

Body System	Side Effects
Lung	Inflammation of the lung/infection (pneumonitis)
	Form scar-like tissue (pulmonary fibrosis) restricting function
	Dry cough
	Shortness of breath
	Fatigue
	Wheezing

The "Chemo Brain" Effect

When chemotherapy treatment ends, some people complain of difficulty in concentrating or remembering daily tasks. Some find themselves having to write down every task they have to do for the day. Usually they can get through the regular daily activities of living, but sometimes they can't do certain activities or tasks that they could do before they had chemotherapy.

This symptom was first reported by breast cancer patients and has come to be called *chemo brain*. Chemo brain has been shown to be caused by not just chemotherapy but other cancer treatments as well, including surgery, radiation, and immunotherapy, which can increase inflammation and impair the immune system that in turn can cause changes in brain function.

When the immune system is impaired, there's an increase in the release of *cytokines* (proteins that send messages between cells) in the brain, which affects brain function. However, a study at City of Hope National Medical Center indicated that chemo brain symptoms were likely caused by the *cancer* increasing the release of cytokines in the brain, not the chemotherapy. The causes of chemo brain continue to be controversial.

Some of the common symptoms seen with chemo brain are as follows:

» Difficulty in coming up with the right word

» Hard to follow a conversation

» Inability to concentrate or focus

» Difficulty in multitasking

» Forgetfulness

>> Loss of math skills

>> Fatigue, lack of energy

>> Confusion or fogginess

Even if you do develop chemo brain, rest assured it's not permanent. And there are strategies you can use to improve your memory and cognitive function. Here's what you can do to help your chemo brain:

>> **Mindfulness:** Participate in yoga and mindfulness/meditation practices to help you develop the skill of paying attention.

>> **Cognitive exercises:** Participate in brain exercises such as word puzzles, math quizzes, or any type of activity or board games such as chess.

>> **Physical exercises:** Your memory and physical function are improved with exercise due to the release of endorphins and reduction in inflammatory processes. However, you must exercise in moderation because you will have fatigue from receiving the chemotherapy.

>> **Asking others for help:** If you have an exam coming up or have a job that is task oriented and will need extra work, ask your oncologist for a letter to submit to the school or employer to accommodate your memory deficit. Don't suffer in silence because of a temporary delay in your memory.

>> **Focusing on strengths, not weaknesses:** Even though your memory is a bit delayed, it doesn't mean you're no longer a great cook or coach. Continue to build on the tasks that you can do well, so that you can be encouraged while your memory recovers.

Understanding the Oncotype DX Test

Oncotype DX is a genomic test. *Genomic* means it's a test involving genes, and groups of genes contain the instructions to make molecules required for life, such as proteins. Oncotype DX is often used by a treatment team, if a tumor is hormone-receptor-positive, to determine whether chemotherapy and hormonal therapies are likely to be beneficial for the breast cancer. This test analyzes the expression of a group of 21 genes within a tumor from a sample removed during surgery. Because cancer cells have mutations and are different than normal cells, the genes made in the tumor cells are distinct from normal cells. The pattern of these genes in your tumor can help indicate its sensitivity to certain chemotherapeutic agents.

There are two different types of Oncotype DX tests — one for patients with DCIS, and one for patients with early breast cancer. There are two main reasons for a doctor to order an Oncotype DX:

>> To determine the risk of recurrence for an early-stage, estrogen-receptor-positive breast cancer, and to see whether chemotherapy would be beneficial after breast cancer surgery.

>> To determine the risk of recurrence for DCIS (ductal carcinoma in situ) and/or the risk of a new invasive cancer in the same breast, and if radiation therapy is beneficial after breast surgery.

REMEMBER

The Oncotype DX test won't be the only deciding factor for your treatment. Your treatment team will combine an evaluation of the Oncotype DX test with your pathology (stage and grade of cancer and receptor status) and other features of the cancer before making a treatment recommendation.

Who should have an Oncotype Dx test?

>> If you are diagnosed with stage I or II invasive breast cancer

>> If your cancer is estrogen-receptor-positive, HER2– (HER2-negative)

>> If you have lymph node negative disease, or are postmenopausal with one to three positive lymph nodes, at the discretion of the oncologist

How does Oncotype DX work?

Oncotype DX is a *prognostic* or predictive genomic test that analyzes the behavior of 21 genes in your tumor, which are distinct from that of normal tissue in your body. Oncotype DX can provide answers to the following questions:

>> How likely is it that the breast cancer will return?

>> How likely are you to benefit from chemotherapy if you're being treated for early-stage invasive breast cancer? This is not commonly used.

>> How likely you are to benefit from radiation therapy if you're being treated for DCIS?

Interpreting the recurrence score

The results of Oncotype DX test in early-stage breast cancer are reported in the form of a *recurrence score* between 0 and 100:

>> **Under 18:** Low risk of cancer recurring. Chemotherapy benefit would likely be small and wouldn't outweigh the potential side effects.

>> **18–30:** Intermediate (moderate) risk of cancer recurring. Chemotherapy benefit is not known.

>> **31 and higher:** High risk of cancer recurrence, and the benefits of chemotherapy are likely to be greater than the risks of side effects.

Understanding the MammaPrint Test

MammaPrint is a genomic test that analyzes 70 genes that are associated with breast cancer metastasis to help determine your biological risk of recurrence. MammaPrint can help answer the following:

>> Who is at risk for recurrence

>> Whether you can safely forgo chemotherapy

>> What the best treatment is for you

Interpreting MammaPrint results

The results of the MammaPrint test are reported as *low risk* or *high risk.* Mamma-Print is used by many oncologists and surgeons in conjunction with other criteria to help determine the treatment plan for breast cancer.

>> **Low risk:** When the MammaPrint result is low risk, it means that you have a low risk of cancer coming back within ten years without any additional treatment after surgery. Therefore, treatment with endocrine or hormonal therapy such as tamoxifen or aromatase inhibitors may often be sufficient treatment after surgery.

>> **High risk:** When the MammaPrint result is high risk, it means that you have a higher risk of cancer coming back within ten years without any additional treatment after surgery. However, you will have the benefit from aggressive treatment, and chemotherapy may be recommended.

TIP

Talk to your cancer doctor about whether Oncotype DX or MammaPrint biomarker testing is right for you. Your doctor may base the decision on a specific practice guideline from institutions such as the National Comprehensive Cancer Network (NCCN) or the American Society of Clinical Oncology (ASCO).

Preparing for Chemotherapy

You will meet with a medical oncologist who is specialized in treating cancers with chemotherapy and hormonal therapy (see Chapter 11 for more on hormonal therapy). The oncologist will prepare your treatment plan. You may receive chemotherapy before or after surgery.

Chemotherapy before surgery: Neoadjuvant chemotherapy

If your tumor is large or you are receptor-positive for HER2, your medical oncologist may recommend chemotherapy before surgery to help shrink the tumor and to find out how sensitive the tumor is to the medication. Having chemotherapy before surgery, as mentioned earlier, is called neoadjuvant chemotherapy.

TIP

If a breast tumor shrinks, that may mean that you will require less surgery. For example, if you had a 5 cm mass in your breast and have a B or C bra cup size, getting chemotherapy before surgery may shrink the tumor to 1 cm, and you may be able to safely have a lumpectomy instead of a mastectomy. Talk to your surgeon and medical oncologist if you have questions about neo adjuvant therapy. After surgery you may need radiation therapy and hormonal therapy.

Chemotherapy after surgery: Adjuvant chemotherapy

Adjuvant chemotherapy is chemotherapy that is given after surgery. Your medical oncologist may recommend adjuvant chemotherapy for the following reasons:

» Lymph nodes under your arm are positive for breast cancer cells.

» Breast tumor was large.

» Breast cancer cells were high grade (grade 3).

» Breast cancer cells did not test positive for hormone receptors (estrogen, progesterone, or HER2) and are likely to not respond well to hormone therapy. Being negative for all three receptors is often called *triple negative breast disease.*

» Cancer cells are at high risk to break away from the breast tumor and spread to other parts of the body. Chemotherapy can kill these cells.

Good Questions to Ask Your Doctor

REMEMBER

If you're unsure or unclear about anything, never hesitate to ask. You have to participate in your treatment, and understanding what is happening is vital. It is important that you ask your doctor about chemotherapy for your breast cancer if that appears to be on the horizon. Here are some good questions to ask:

» Why are you recommending chemotherapy for me?

» Is there any other treatment I can have instead? Why or why not?

» What is the goal of the chemotherapy treatment? Cure or palliative?

» What medicines will I be taking and will I have any input about the type of chemotherapy I get?

» What are the short- and long-term side effects of the chemotherapy?

» I know that chemotherapy may make my hair fall out. Is there any other treatment that won't make my hair fall out?

» Is there any treatment that won't make me infertile?

» Will I be able to meet a fertility specialist to freeze the eggs from the ovaries before I start chemotherapy treatment?

» How will chemotherapy affect my immune system, and should I take anything to help boost my immune system?

» How long will my course of chemotherapy treatment take?

» What can I do to help alleviate side effects during chemotherapy?

» How will I know if I get an infection?

» Do I need time off from work while receiving chemotherapy treatment?

» Is there a number I can call to speak to someone in your team anytime I experience new symptoms or have concerns?

» Who can I contact for emotional support?

Chapter **11**

Endocrine, Biological, and Cutting-Edge Therapies

E ndocrine therapy (ET), also known as *hormonal therapy*, for breast cancer is different from hormone-replacement therapy. Some hormone-replacement therapies provide a synthetic or biological form of hormones (for example, estrogen, testosterone, or progesterone), which are normally produced in the body naturally, for relief of post menopausal symptoms such as hot flashes, vaginal dryness, mood swings, and so on. That's different from the hormonal therapy used in the treatment of breast cancer.

Breast cancer research in recent years has also developed biological and antiHER2 therapies for treatment of breast cancers that have a high risk of coming back and for advanced disease (stage IV) in combination with chemotherapy. Biological therapy has also been used to treat bone-marrow suppression or low blood count caused by chemotherapy.

Breast cancer treatment has come a long way, but there is no one-size-fits-all treatment. It's more like a puzzle that's placed together with various types of medication aiming for a cure or for increasing the chances of survival.

Endocrine Therapy in the Treatment of Breast Cancer

Hormonal therapy, as mentioned, is often called *endocrine* therapy. The endocrine system is made of glands that produce and secrete hormones. Because endocrine therapy used for breast cancer targets the hormone estrogen that is normally present in our bodies, these terms are used interchangeably. Estrogen can promote the development of breast cancer, and hormonal therapy involves the use of oral medications that decrease or prevent the production of estrogen, or block estrogen receptors to keep estrogen away from breast cells. Endocrine therapy medicines are used to achieve the following:

>> Lower the risk of estrogen-receptor-positive breast cancer coming back

>> Lower the risk of estrogen-receptor-positive breast cancer in individuals who are at high risk for developing breast cancer in the future

>> Help shrink or slow the growth of *advanced-stage* or *metastatic* estrogen-receptor-positive breast cancers

Endocrine therapy may be recommended for 5–10 years only if your breast cancer cells tested positive for *estrogen receptors* (ER+), cells that have a special receptor protein that binds to the estrogen hormone. ER+ cancer cells may need estrogen to grow, and may die or stop growing with a substance that blocks the action or blocks the binding of estrogen. *Progesterone-receptor-positive* (PR+) cancer cells are cells that have a special receptor protein that binds to the progesterone hormone. PR+ cancer cells may need progesterone to grow, and may die or stop growing when an anti-progesterone agent is used. See Chapter 5 for more on the terms ER+/PR+.

There are three types of endocrine therapy used for breast cancer prevention:

>> Selective estrogen-receptor modulators (SERMs), also called *antiestrogens*:

- Tamoxifen (marketed as Nolvadex)

- Raloxifene (marketed as Evista)

- Toremifene citrate (marketed as Fareston)

» Aromatase inhibitors:

- Anastrozole (marketed as Arimidex)

- Exemestane (marketed as Aromasin)

- Letrozole (marketed as Femara)

» Selective estrogen-receptor downregulators, called SERDs:

- Fulvestrant (marketed as Faslodex)

Side effects of endocrine therapy

REMEMBER

Everyone reacts differently to medications, and you may have more or fewer side effects than others. Overall, side effects can usually be controlled and often improve over time as your body gets use to the medications. Some side effects are experienced with all types of hormone therapies, whereas others are specific to a type of medication. Table 11-1 shows many common side effects of each kind of medicine.

TABLE 11-1 **Common Side Effects of Endocrine Therapies**

	Aromatase Inhibitors			SERMs			ERDs
	Arimidex	Aromasin	Femara	Tamoxifen	Evista	Fareston	Faslodex
Bone/joint pain	*	*	*		*	*	
Bone thinning	*	*	*				
Osteoporosis	*	*	*				
Hot flashes	*	*	*	*	*	*	*
Fatigue	*	*	*	*			
Weakness	*	*					
Headache		*		*			*
Blood clots				*	*		
Weight gain			*				
Insomnia		*			*		
Increased sweating					*	*	
Dizziness			*				

(continued)

TABLE 11-1 *(continued)*

	Aromatase Inhibitors			SERMs			ERDs
	Arimidex	Aromasin	Femara	Tamoxifen	Evista	Fareston	Faslodex
Drowsiness			*				
Endometrial cancer				*		*	
Mood swings				*		*	
Hair thinning	*	*	*	*			
Dry skin				*	*	*	
Rash						*	
Loss of libido				*			
Vaginal discharge or bleeding						*	
Vision problems						*	
Back pain							*
Stomach or abdominal pain							*
Hypercalcemia						*	
Leg cramps					*		
Swelling					*	*	
Depression				*			
Stroke				*	*		
Higher cholesterol			*				
Flu-like symptoms					*		

Preparing for Endocrine Therapy

First, you will meet with a medical oncologist who is specialized in treating cancers with hormonal therapy. There are two main kinds of hormonal therapy: therapy given before surgery (called *neoadjuvant* therapy) and therapy given after surgery (called *adjuvant* therapy).

Endocrine therapy before surgery

Your medical oncologist may give you hormonal therapy to shrink a large or locally advanced breast cancer before surgery. This treatment is only given to women with estrogen-receptor-positive breast cancer. The goal is to shrink the tumor so that the breast can be conserved by having the cancer removed with a lumpectomy or wide local excision instead of a mastectomy.

Your medical oncologist will continue to monitor the size of the breast tumor while administering hormonal therapy. This will help them to determine whether the treatment is working and whether to continue treatment or recommend immediate surgery. Your doctor will take your individual situation into account when deciding which treatment may suit you best.

Endocrine therapy after surgery

Hormonal therapy is often given after breast surgery, after radiation therapy has been completed or chemotherapy has ended. It's been proven to reduce the risk of breast cancer coming back as well as prevent a new breast cancer from developing. Hormonal therapy is usually given for five to ten years. Your medical oncologist will determine the best length of treatment for you.

If you can't have surgery

Sometimes breast surgery may not be an option for you. Such a case may be related to having significant health problems, for example, that can increase your risk for surgical complications. Or you may not want to have surgery. Your oncology specialists may offer you hormonal therapy if your receptors are positive for estrogen and progesterone. Sometimes this is called *primary endocrine therapy.* Primary ET won't get rid of the cancer but it may stop it from growing or may shrink it for several months or up to a few years. If the cancer starts to grow again, you may need other types of treatment.

Asking plenty of questions

It's important for you to ask your doctor about endocrine therapy for your breast cancer. Some of the questions you can ask include the following:

>> Why are you recommending endocrine therapy for me?

>> Is there any other treatment I can have in addition to or instead of endocrine therapy?

>> What is the goal of the endocrine therapy?

>> What medicines will I take and can I choose the type of medicines?

>> What are the short- and long-term side effects of endocrine therapy?

>> Is there any treatment that won't make me infertile?

>> How long will my course of treatment take for endocrine therapy?

>> What can I do to help with side effects during endocrine therapy?

>> How will I know if I get an infection?

>> Do I need time off from work while receiving treatment?

>> Is there a number I can call to speak to someone in your team anytime I experience new symptoms or have concerns?

>> Whom can I contact for emotional support?

Biological or Targeted Therapy in the Treatment of Breast Cancer

Biological therapies, or *targeted* therapies, are treatments given to interrupt the cancer cell function or processes. These therapies may do the following:

>> Stop cancer cells from growing

>> Identify cancer cells and kill them

>> Increase the immune system's attack on the cancer cells

Biological therapy is recommended based on the following:

>> The type of breast cancer you have

>> How far your breast cancer has spread (which stage you are in)

>> Prior cancer treatments you have had

TIP

Although many biological therapies for cancer are still experimental, some have proven to be very effective in treating breast cancer.

Biological therapies for breast cancer stop cancer cells from signaling or change the way cells interact to make them stop dividing and growing. These targeted therapies involve medications that target specific protein molecules on cancer cells. Monoclonal antibodies, cyclin-dependent kinase inhibitors, tyrosine kinase inhibitors, mammalian target of rapamycin (mTOR) inhibitors, and PARP inhibitors are some types of targeted therapies used in the treatment of breast cancer.

Monoclonal antibodies, for example, identify and attach to specific protein receptors on the cell that make the cancer grow. The antibodies attach to these proteins and help stop growth signals in the cancer cells, which can keep them from multiplying and spreading. Monoclonal antibodies may also be used with chemotherapy as adjuvant therapy.

HER2 is a target for biological therapy in breast cancer. Approximately 15–18 percent of newly diagnosed individuals with breast cancer have an abundance of HER2 receptors, and this causes breast cancer cells to grow faster. If your breast cancer is found to have an abundance of HER2+ receptors on your biopsy, you may be given trastuzumab (Herceptin). Trastuzumab is a biological therapy that blocks HER2. See Chapter 7 for more on the HER2 receptor, including an illustration.

WARNING

Having HER2+ breast cancer means the cancer is more aggressive and that it can grow faster and spread quickly to other parts of the body. But the good news is that there is a targeted therapy to help kill these types of cancer cells.

Types of biological therapies

Any treatment that uses your body's natural immune defenses to ward off infection, fight a disease, or protect the body from a side effect of treatment is called a *biological* therapy. This section discusses biological therapies.

Monoclonal antibodies

>> Trastuzumab (Herceptin) blocks the effects of the protein growth factor on the HER2, which sends growth signals to breast cancer cells, thus stopping the growth of breast cancer cells. Herceptin is the most widely used among the monoclonal antibodies — we talk more about it shortly.

>> Pertuzumab (Perjeta) is usually given along with trastuzumab and chemotherapy to treat breast cancer for certain individuals with HER2+ breast cancer that has spread to other parts of the body. It is also used to treat early stage HER2+ breast cancer.

>> Ado-trastuzumab emtansine (Kadcyla) is a combination of an antibody and a cancer medication that is used to treat breast cancers that have spread to other parts of the body or have come back.

TIP

Trastuzumab (Herceptin) may be given along with chemotherapy or given before or after surgery and radiation.

Tyrosine kinase inhibitors

Tyrosine kinase inhibitors are targeted therapies that block signals that are needed for tumors to grow and may be used with other anti-cancer drugs as adjuvant therapy. Tyrosine kinase inhibitors include Lapatinib (Tykerb), which blocks the effects of the HER2 protein and other proteins inside tumor cells. It's often given in combination with other drugs to treat patients with HER2+ breast cancer that was not controlled after receiving trastuzumab.

Cyclin-dependent kinase inhibitors

Cyclin-dependent kinase inhibitors block proteins called *cyclin-dependent kinases*, which cause the growth of cancer cells. Cyclin-dependent kinase inhibitors include palbociclib and ribociclib, which is used with the medication letrozole to treat breast cancer that is ER+ and HER2− and that has spread to other parts of the body. It's used in postmenopausal women whose cancer was not treated previously with hormone therapy. Palbociclib is sometimes used with fulvestrant in women whose breast cancer has progressed after treatment with hormone therapy.

Mammalian target of rapamycin (mTOR) inhibitors

Mammalian target of rapamycin (mTOR) inhibitors block the mTOR protein, which may prevent cancer cells from growing and prevent new growth of blood vessels that tumors need to survive. mTOR inhibitors include everolimus, which is given to postmenopausal women with hormone-receptor-positive advanced stage breast cancer that is also HER2− and that has not improved with other treatment.

PARP inhibitors

PARP inhibitors are a type of targeted therapy that stops DNA repair, which may cause the cancer cells to die. PARP inhibitors has been shown to be effective in treating cancers that have known positive BRCA mutation status. For example, olaparib (Lynparza) is the first PARP inhibitor that has been approved by the FDA for BRCA-mutated ovarian cancer because of the success seen with the drug in clinical trials. The recent report from the phase III OLYMPIAN trial showed olaparib to improve progression-free survival more than standard chemotherapy in BRCA-positive breast cancer. Now we can look towards the FDA approval of olaparib for BRCA-positive breast cancer in the future.

Trastuzumab and pertuzumab: Monoclonal antibodies

Herceptin should not be given to individuals who are pregnant or have the following heart problems:

>> Chest pain or angina that requires medication

>> Congestive heart failure

>> Uncontrolled blood pressure

>> Heart valve disease that causes symptoms

>> Uncontrolled atrial fibrillation or other abnormal heart rhythms

Prior to starting Herceptin treatment, your oncology team will test your heart with an echocardiogram, which is a noninvasive nuclear medicine test that enables clinicians to obtain information about heart muscle activity every three months while receiving treatment to determine whether Herceptin is causing problems.

Common side effects of Herceptin include the following (at least 10 out of every 100 patients may have these effects):

>> Reaction to the medication while it's given (infusion reaction)

>> Increased risk of infection

>> Tiredness and weakness (fatigue)

>> Soreness at the injection site if Herceptin is given as an injection

>> Diarrhea

>> Skin rash

>> Taste changes

>> Loss of appetite

>> Easy bruising

>> Sore, red eyes (conjunctivitis)

>> Numbness or tingling in fingers or toes

>> Difficulty sleeping

>> Hot flashes

Rarer side effects include the following (at least 1 out of every 100 patients may have these effects):

>> **Liver problems:** Having irregular liver function blood tests

>> **Chronic/long-term lung problems:** Causing difficulty in breathing

>> **Amenorrhea:** Women no longer have a menstrual cycle temporarily

>> **Loss of fertility:** You may not be able to get pregnant or father a child

REMEMBER

Side effects of Herceptin can be mild or severe and may improve or worsen while on treatment. New side effects can develop as treatment continues. Which side effects you may get depends on

>> Your general health status.

>> The dose of the medication you receive.

>> How often you have had the medication before.

Talk to your oncology team if you experience any side effects from the medication so they can help to manage the symptoms and provide education and reassurance.

Immunotherapy and Cancer Vaccines

When you see the word *immunotherapy*, you automatically think about the immune system or the part of the body that is able to fight against bacteria, viruses, or diseases. You are so right. In a cancer patient, the immune system has T-cells and cancer cells that produce certain proteins, and these proteins can prevent T-cells from killing cancer cells. Some of the (checkpoint) proteins found on T-cells or cancer cells include PD-1/PD-L1 and CTLA-4/B7-1/B7-2. The *immune checkpoint inhibitor* is a type of drug that blocks these proteins made by T-cells and cancer cells. When these proteins are blocked, the T-cells are able to kill the cancer cells more effectively. Some immune checkpoint inhibitors are used in combination with cancer vaccines to enhance the anticancer immune system response to treatment. Currently, several ongoing clinical trials are focused on the use of immune checkpoint therapies to treat breast cancer by targeting CTLA-4, PD-1, or lymphocyte activation gene-3 (LAG-3) pathways.

Cancer vaccines

Traditionally, vaccines prevent the development of a disease (for example, the MMR vaccine you are given as a child that prevents measles, mumps, and rubella). Scientists around the world are actively researching vaccines to prevent and treat common forms of cancer. Gardasil was the first FDA-approved vaccine to prevent cancer. It was developed from antigens found in the HPV (human papilloma) virus. Prevention of infection with certain types of HPV can prevent the development of cervical cancer later in life.

Cancer vaccines contain specific *antigens* (small molecules commonly found on cancer cells) to enhance your immune system's ability to recognize and respond to cancer by stimulating immune cells such as the B-cell, a type of white blood cell that makes antibodies. B-cells are part of the immune system and develop from stem cells in the bone marrow. A killer T-cell is a type of immune cell that can kill certain cells, including foreign cells, cancer cells, and cells infected with a virus. Killer T-cells can be separated from other blood cells, grown in the laboratory, and given to a patient to kill cancer cells. A killer T-cell is a type of white blood cell and a type of lymphocyte.

Cancer treatment vaccines

Cancer treatment vaccines are the wave of the future. Many academic centers around the world are engaging in clinical trials and various treatments for specific cancers. Cancer treatment vaccines are designed to treat cancers that have already developed, rather than prevent them in the first place. Cancer treatment vaccines contain cancer-associated antigens to enhance the immune system's response to a patient's tumor cells. The cancer-associated antigens can be proteins or another type of molecule found on the surface of or inside cancer cells that can stimulate immune cells (B-cells or killer T-cells) to attack them.

The making of a cancer vaccine

The cancer prevention vaccines that are approved by the FDA are produced using antigens from microbes — for example, HPV, a type of virus that can cause abnormal tissue growth (for example, warts) and other changes to cells. Infection for a long time with certain types of HPV can cause cervical cancer. HPV may also play a role in some other types of cancer, such as anal, vaginal, vulvar, penile, oropharyngeal, and squamous cell skin cancers. HBV, also called *hepatitis B virus*, is a virus that causes hepatitis (inflammation of the liver). It is carried and passed to others through the blood and other body fluids. Different ways the virus can spread include sharing needles with an infected person and being stuck accidentally by a needle contaminated with the virus. Infants born to infected mothers may also become infected with the virus. Although many patients who are infected with HBV may not have symptoms, long-term infection may lead to cirrhosis (scarring of the liver) and liver cancer. The antigens are proteins, and they make up the outer shell of the virus. Only a part of the microbe is used in the vaccine development, which results in cancer vaccines not being infectious or causing disease.

Some researchers are making cancer vaccines by developing synthetic versions of the antigen that mimics the function of the original antigen found on the cancer cell. Through this type of development, the chemical structure of the synthetic antigen is made to have a stronger response to the original antigen and a greater effect on killing the cancer cell. Types of antigens that are used in the manufacturing of cancer vaccines are carbohydrates (sugars), proteins, gangliosides (carbohydrate-lipid combination), and glycoproteins or glycopeptides (carbohydrate-protein combinations).

Cancer vaccines are also being made with killed or weakened cancer cells that have specific cancer-associated antigens on the cell surface. These cells may come from a patient and be given back in the form of the vaccine (called *autologous* vaccine) or from another patient (called *allogenic* vaccine).

These cancer vaccines are approved by the FDA for different cancers:

>> **Sipuleucel-T (brand name Provenge):** FDA-approved for men with prostate cancer. It stimulates an immune system attack on prostatic acid phosphatase (PAP), an antigen commonly found on prostate cancer cells.

>> **Talimogene laherparepvec (T-VEC):** FDA-approved oncolytic virus therapy, for the treatment of metastatic melanoma.

The following immune checkpoint inhibitors are approved by the FDA for different types of cancers:

>> **Keytruda (pembrolizumab):** FDA-approved for the treatment of a type of bladder and urinary tract cancer called *urothelial carcinoma.*

>> **Bavencio (avelumab):** FDA-approved for the treatment of metastatic Merkel cell carcinoma, a rare and aggressive skin cancer.

>> **Opdivo (nivolumab):** FDA-approved for treatment of metastatic non-small cell lung cancer, metastatic melanoma, advanced renal cell carcinoma, recurrent or metastatic squamous cell carcinoma, classical Hodgkin lymphoma (cHL), and previously treated locally advanced or metastatic urothelial carcinoma.

>> **Imfinzi (durvalumab):** FDA-approved for the treatment of bladder cancer and locally advanced or metastatic urothelial carcinoma in patients whose disease continued to progress despite treatment with neoadjuvant or adjuvant chemotherapy.

Some cancer vaccines show limited toxicity and very few side effects. Current clinical trials are using them in combination with chemotherapy, radiation, hormonal therapy, and targeted therapies. Sometimes cancer vaccines are used in combination with a drug that helps change the way the immune cells interact using PD-1, a protein in humans that is encoded by the PDCD1 gene. PD-1 is a cell surface receptor that is expressed on immune cells (T-cells and B-cells) and binds two *ligands* (a molecule that binds to another, usually larger molecule). Nivolumab (Opdivo) is one of those drugs and is a monoclonal antibody that blocks PD-1. When you block PD-1 on T-cells (also on some tumor cells), it can no longer bind to PD-L1 (its ligand, or binding partner), which can result in suppression of T-cell activation. Nivolumab (Opdivo) is FDA-approved for use in treating advanced renal cell cancer, metastatic melanoma, metastatic non-small cell lung cancer, recurrent or metastatic squamous cell cancer, and metastatic urothelial cancer. It blocks PD-1, and this allows your body's immune system to attack cancer cells.

TIP

There are 24 active NIH clinical trials with breast cancer patients currently taking place. The future is promising for immunotherapy for breast cancer treatment.

Cancer vaccine side effects

The following are the more common side effects of cancer vaccines:

>> **Site of injection:** Inflammation that includes swelling, redness, pain, warming of the skin, rash, and itchiness.

>> **Flu-like symptoms:** These may include fever, chills, dizziness, headaches, weakness, nausea, vomiting, fatigue, muscle ache, and occasional shortness of breath.

>> **Elevated blood pressure:** This is an indicator that the body is responding to the cancer vaccine.

Here are some uncommon side effects of cancer vaccines:

>> Asthma

>> Pelvic inflammatory disease

>> Appendicitis

>> Autoimmune disease (for example, rheumatoid arthritis, systemic lupus erythematosus, and Reynard's)

WARNING

Vaccines that are made with microbes (such as sipuleucel-T) can cause infection at the injection site or blood in the urine.

Precision Medicine

Even though we have biological therapies that include targeted therapy, monoclonal antibodies, and immunotherapies, cancer has become so complex that many of these treatments don't work for every person.

Breast cancer research is constantly evolving into new treatments, especially in the area of *precision* medicine or *personalized* medicine. Precision medicine in cancer therapy is the use of a person's genetic information to treat or diagnose their disease. From everything we know about the development of cancer, it's a disease of the genome because it carries its own set of mutations at the cell DNA level. If we understand the genetic changes within a cancer cell, we're better armed to develop tailored therapies that target specific biomarkers in a patient's genetic profile.

Benefits of precision medicine

Benefits of precision medicine include the following:

>> Less drug resistance due to therapies that will target the specific genetic changes within the tumor of an individual

>> The ability to predict which medication will be more effective in a specific breast cancer of a patient

>> A large data depository of information on many cancers according to their DNA changes that matches evidence-proven treatments

Emerging Therapies

There is a constant effort by researchers to find new treatments for various types of breast cancer. New clinical trials are developing all the time in various populations with different ethnicities and risk factors to help find a permanent cure or more effective treatment for breast cancer. The results of clinical trials are the foundation for establishing guidelines for breast cancer treatment. The following sections discuss the discoveries in targeted therapy and cell signaling that are emerging treatments for breast cancer.

Targeted therapy: Immunoliposomes

Researchers at the University of California San Francisco's Comprehensive Cancer Center are using a new technology called *immunoliposomes* to kill cancer cells. An immunoliposome is a molecule that consist of a fat (lipid) ball that contains a chemotherapy agent. An antibody is used to identify the protein marker on the surface of the cancer cell and then deliver the fat ball into the cancer cell, where the chemotherapy agent is released and the cancer cell dies. The benefit of a treatment like this is that the chemotherapy would not be delivered in high concentrations to the noncancerous tissue in the body, resulting (in theory) in fewer side effects to the normal tissues.

Cell signaling

The communication activity within a cell is quite noisy — cells are constantly sending and receiving messages to and from each other. Some cells send messages to stimulate growth, whereas others send messages to stop growth or to destroy and cause cell death. Any type of cell-signaling process involves protein markers that are on the surface of cells and the genes that are contained within the cells. When the cell-signaling process is regulated, normal cell growth and proliferation occurs. When the cell-signaling process goes out of control, then cells are growing rapidly and changing in shape and function, leading to cancers. This process is called *deregulation* of the cell.

Researchers are currently working on identifying genes that can stop deregulation of breast tissue. This process will involve identifying the faulty genes that cause the cell to malfunction and target either the upstream or the downstream signaling process with medications.

Chapter **12**

Breast Reconstruction

Many women may choose to have breast reconstruction surgery when they have breast cancer or later, but breast reconstruction may not be right for everyone. *Breast reconstruction* is surgery to make a new breast after removal of the entire breast or part of the breast. The goal of breast reconstruction is to make a breast of similar size and shape to your natural breast. They won't be identical. However, your breasts can be made almost identical when you have both breasts removed due to high breast cancer risk.

Women may choose breast reconstruction for the following reasons:

» To regain the shape of their natural breast

» To ensure that their chest appears balanced when wearing a bra or form-fitted top

» To avoid wearing a breast prosthesis (or breast form) that fits inside a bra

» To feel good about themselves and maintain a good self-image

WARNING

Breast reconstruction can leave scars, which can often fade over time. Plastic surgeons are using newer techniques to reduce scarring as well as to fade the scar.

Breast reconstruction after a mastectomy can make you feel better about how you look and renew your self-confidence. But keep in mind that the reconstructed breast won't be a perfect match and can't substitute for your natural breast. If tissue from your tummy, shoulder, or buttocks will be used as part of the reconstruction, those areas will also look different after surgery. Talk with your surgeon about surgical scars and changes in shape or contour. Ask where they will be and how they will look and feel after they heal.

Breast plastic surgeons specialize in breast augmentation, reducing scarring or disfigurement that may occur as a result of treatment for diseases. The reconstruction of a breast can be done in several ways, depending on whether part of the breast or the entire natural breast will be removed.

Figure 12-1 illustrates a bilateral mastectomy.

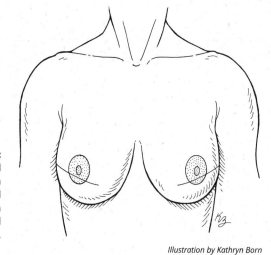

FIGURE 12-1:
Bilateral mastectomy with delayed reconstruction and tattooed nipple.

Illustration by Kathryn Born

When Should You Have Breast Reconstruction?

Breast reconstruction can be done at the same time as the breast cancer surgery (called *immediate* reconstruction). It can also be done in a two-stage process where tissue expander (a temporary placeholder) is placed at the time of breast cancer surgery. For the final breast reconstruction, a synthetic implant or tissue from another part of your body is used to complete the procedure at a later date. You can also have breast reconstruction after breast cancer surgery, called *delayed* reconstruction.

Your breast plastic surgeon will consider the following before making a recommendation for your breast reconstruction surgery.

>> Type and stage of your breast cancer

>> Additional treatments that you might need for your breast cancer

>> Your body shape

>> Your feelings

>> Your personal preferences and lifestyle

When you meet with your breast plastic surgeon, she will discuss your reconstructive options, including the risks, benefits, and options available for each procedure. You'll also discuss the expected cosmetic outcomes from the reconstruction.

Immediate breast reconstruction

An immediate reconstruction is typically recommended when you have no known breast cancer in the breast, and it gives you a new breast straight away. For example, when women have pre-cancerous lesions removed or when women with positive BRCA mutation who have not yet developed cancer have their breast removed (called a *prophylactic mastectomy*), they may have immediate reconstructive surgery reconstruction. Even though the breast is not identical to the one that was removed, most women find that immediate reconstruction helps them cope better with the loss of a breast.

When you do have breast cancer, you will have delayed reconstruction because it gives time for the final surgery pathology to determine whether you have *clear margins* (that is, no cancer cells are seen at the outer edge of the tissue that was removed). If you are found to have positive margins, or cancer cells are seen at the outer edge of the tissue, then an additional surgery may be indicated to remove the cancer cells. Having had immediate reconstruction would interfere with the surgery in this case.

Advantages

>> You will have your newly reconstructed breast after waking up from your lumpectomy or mastectomy. Immediate breast reconstruction may also have a psychological benefit, as you won't have a period of time with "no breasts."

>> You will have fewer surgeries and fewer anesthetics.

>> Your reconstructed breasts may form better because the plastic surgeon can use the extra skin that's already there, leading to improved cosmetic outcome.

>> You may have less scarring on the reconstructed breast itself.

>> It involves lower healthcare costs.

Disadvantages

>> You may not have as much time to decide on the type of breast reconstruction that you want.

>> If you're having radiation therapy after surgery, it may cause injury to the reconstructed breast.

>> Difficulty in detecting mastectomy skin problems.

>> Your doctor may advise you not to have implant reconstruction if you're having radiation therapy afterwards. However, you may have a temporary implant during radiation with another breast reconstruction surgery after radiation has completed.

>> You will have longer hospitalization and recovery times than if you had mastectomy alone.

>> Complications from breast reconstruction surgery may delay chemotherapy that you need. Chemotherapy stops the body from being able to heal well, so if you have any problems with wound healing after your breast reconstruction, you won't be able to start chemotherapy until the problems have been resolved. If you were given chemotherapy at this time, it would stop the wound healing and cause a serious infection.

Research has shown that the most benefit received from chemotherapy is when it is given within six weeks of breast cancer surgery. And if your breast reconstruction surgery causes delayed wound healing, then chemotherapy could be delayed beyond those six weeks.

Immediate breast reconstruction requires a lot of coordination between the breast surgeon and plastic surgeon operating room (OR) schedules, because they both will have to be in the OR at the same time, along with other members of the team to ensure the success of the procedure.

TIP

Immediate breast reconstruction may be a good option if you have the following:

>> Smaller tumor size (less than 2 cm)

>> Low chance of needing radiation therapy after surgery

>> Diagnosis of a non invasive cancer or pre-cancer (such as ADH or DCIS)

>> Auxiliary lymph nodes under your armpit don't have cancer

>> Clear margins from surgery

>> You're healthy to undergo general anesthetic

>> Prophylactic (preventive) mastectomy due to having a genetic mutation (such as BRCA 1 or 2)

Delayed breast reconstruction

Some women prefer to get over the mastectomy and breast cancer treatment first, before they think about reconstruction. Delayed reconstruction is typically done after the mastectomy site has healed. Healing can take six months or even several years after the mastectomy.

Advantages

>> You have more time to look at all types of reconstruction options and discuss them with your plastic surgeon.

>> If you're having additional cancer treatment after mastectomy (such as radiation), it won't cause problems at the reconstruction site.

>> You schedule the surgery at your leisure or at the time you elected.

Disadvantages

>> You have a period after the mastectomy during which you have no breast tissue, but you can choose to wear a false breast.

>> You will have a mastectomy scar on the chest wall, which is a larger scar on the reconstructed breast than after immediate reconstruction.

>> Delayed reconstruction requires additional surgery and recovery time.

>> The breast is sometimes difficult to reconstruct after scarring occurs.

TIP

Delayed reconstruction may be a good option if you have the following:

>> Larger breast tumor (over 2 cm)

>> Tumor-free from breast cancer (all cancer was successfully removed in your first surgery) and have completed chemotherapy/radiation therapy

>> Healthy to undergo general anesthesia

>> Radiation therapy completed at least six months prior to surgery

Having both breasts removed

Sometimes the option to remove both breasts is based on the disease, and some-times it's based on the disease plus a patient's anxiety. The guidelines do state that if you have left breast cancer, you can have a lumpectomy with radiation or a mastectomy. Yet often women choose to remove both breasts to reduce the risk of getting another breast cancer. Breast reconstruction options for the non-breast cancer side are the same for a breast cancer side. Here are some possible reasons for removing the other breast when there is no cancer:

>> Breast cancer gene mutation carriers (BRCA1, BRCA2, and so on)

>> Strong family history of breast cancer

>> The original cancer was not found by mammograms or other tests

>> Personal choice of a woman after considering her breast cancer risk

Advantages

>> Easier to have both breasts look the same or symmetric

>> One surgery and one hospital stay

>> Reduced chance of getting breast cancer

>> No need for future mammograms (if all tissue from both breasts is removed)

Disadvantages

>> If abdominal flaps are being used, only half the abdominal tissue can be used for each breast (which limits the size of the reconstructed breasts). Implants, tissue expanders, or back tissue may be needed to make the breasts the right size.

>> Lengthy surgery compared to reconstructing one breast

>> Increased risk for complications

Methods of Breast Reconstruction

There are three methods of breast reconstruction:

>> **Breast implant reconstruction:** This involves removing the whole breast and skin, and using an implant underneath the remaining skin.

>> **Autologous breast reconstruction:** This is reconstruction using your own tissue. It means removing the whole breast, leaving most of the skin, and using tissue from another part of your body to reconstruct the breast.

>> **Combination:** This is reconstruction using your own tissue combined with an implant — a combination of the two previous methods. This can be done when there's not enough of the patient's own tissue to achieve the desired breast size. Often, thin patients with little body fat do not have enough of their own tissue to create full breast flaps.

Breast implant reconstruction

Breast implant reconstruction is popular because it's often used to increase the size of the natural breast when there is no disease while not having to use tissue from another part of your body. There are two types of implants: saline-filled and silicone gel-filled. Both types of implants are manufactured in various shapes, sizes, and profiles.

Both saline and silicone implants are safe and effective.

Breast implant reconstruction can be done as a single-stage process or two-stage process.

Two-stage process

In the two-stage process, the breast shape is first created by placing a tissue expander under the skin and muscle of the chest. A *tissue expander* is a temporary implant that can be infused with saline over time to help stretch the skin out. Remember that the breast tissue and skin were removed by the mastectomy. The tissue expander is gradually inflated over weeks with saline injections to stretch the remaining skin and chest muscle before inserting the permanent breast implant. The expansion process can take six to eight visits over several weeks. Then surgery to exchange the tissue expander for a permanent implant is done after 12–24 weeks. The reconstructed breast is modeled into the final breast shape.

In addition to this surgery, your breast plastic surgeon can reduce or lift the opposite breast at the same time for symmetry, if you desire. Be sure to discuss this with your surgeon prior to the surgery.

Single-stage process

In the single-stage process, the breast tissue and skin are removed by mastectomy, and the plastic surgeon places an adjustable implant under the skin and muscle — similar to a tissue expander — and fills the device over time with saline. The adjustable implant is designed to be permanent.

When the ideal volume is achieved, the plastic surgeon can remove the fill tube and close the internal valve, leaving the device as the permanent implant. This can be done in a clinic setting.

In single-stage implant reconstruction, the breast implant is often placed under the muscle of the chest and then secured in place with a material called *acellular dermal matrix* (ADM). ADM is also known as Alloderm or Allomax. ADM is made from the human skin of donated cadavers, specially prepared for your body to accept it. There are no reports of infection caused by ADM.

REMEMBER

Your breast surgeon will help you determine which implant is best for your body shape or structure.

Advantages include the following:

>> One surgery, one general anesthesia, and one recovery period

>> Fewer scars

>> Satisfactory contour or shape in clothing

Disadvantages include the following:

>> Need frequent office visits for complete tissue expansion

>> Two-stage procedure of tissue expander followed by exchange for permanent implant

>> Difficulty forming nipple projection with nipple reconstruction, due to thinner skin

>> Difficult to achieve similar shape with the natural breast

>> Need to replace implants periodically, which means more surgery

Saline vs. silicone breast implants

Both saline and silicone breast implants have an outer silicone shell; the difference is in the solution that is within the implant. Saline breast implants are empty when they are first placed during surgery and then later filled with sterile saltwater. They are offered to women 18 and older for breast augmentation and at any age for breast reconstruction.

Silicone breast implants are pre-filled with silicone gel — a thick, sticky fluid that closely mimics the feel of human fat when placed during surgery. Most women feel that silicone breast implants feel more like natural breast tissue. They are offered to women 22 and older for breast augmentation and any age for breast reconstruction.

Risks of breast implants

Some of the risks of implants include the following:

>> Scar tissue inside the breast, around the implant, that may change the shape of the breast implant (capsular contracture) — very common, but usually takes years (even a decade) to develop

>> Infection

>> Breast pain

>> Changes in nipple and breast sensation, usually temporary

>> Implant leakage or rupture

Correcting any of these complications might require additional surgery, either to remove or replace the implants.

Autologous breast reconstruction

When you use your own tissue from your body to create the breast, it's called *autologous* tissue. This kind of breast reconstruction uses the patient's own tissue to create a breast mound. This method can create a natural-appearing and durable result in comparison to implant reconstruction. Complete reconstruction of the breast can be accomplished in a one-stage process.

In this method, abdominal tissue is used to reconstruct the breast through transferring the tissue to the chest in the following two ways:

>> **Pedicle transverse rectus abdominis myocutaneous (TRAM) flap:** The rectus muscle (the "abs" or "six-pack") is used as the *flap* (tissue relocated on the body) because it has its own blood supply that protrudes through to the lower abdominal skin and fat. The muscle, along with the fat and skin, can be dissected and relocated to the breast. A tunnel is made under the skin between the abdomen and the mastectomy cavity to relocate the abdominal flap to the chest. The abdominal donor site is closed using either sutures or a strong artificial material (mesh) to reinforce the strength of the abdomen. This

will also give you a "tummy tuck" or *abdominoplasty* at the same time as the breast reconstruction.

> » **Free deep inferior epigastric perforator (DIEP) flap (completely removed and then microsurgically reattached):** This method is an advancement from the pedicled TRAM flap where the rectus muscle is not removed but only the skin and the fat are used to re-create the breast. This procedure requires microsurgical expertise because the lower abdominal tissue must be completely detached from the body and transferred to the chest. Microsurgery allows for the microcirculation to be restored to the transplanted skin and fat.

Advantages of DIEP autologous breast reconstruction include the following:

> » Little to no rectus muscle is disturbed during the process, and the abdominal muscle strength is preserved. This reduces the risk of abdominal hernia.

> » The abdominal flap is completely removed and reattached to the blood vessels in the chest, which provide better blood supply to the reconstructed breast.

Disadvantages include the following:

> » Microsurgery has a 1–3 percent failure rate when reestablishing blood connection to the abdominal tissue transferred to the chest. If this occurs, then reconstruction has failed, and the transferred tissue can't be stored or saved. Another method of breast reconstruction may be considered later in the future.

> » Women who have a history of diabetes, clotting disorders, are active smokers, or are obese are at greater risk for microsurgery failure.

> » The duration of surgery for breast reconstruction microsurgery is usually twice as long as the TRAM flap technique.

Although both methods result in similar breast and abdominal scars, there are some major differences between them.

Autologous tissue with implant reconstruction

This type of breast reconstruction uses both a smaller implant and the patient's natural tissue. If the tissue from the abdomen can't be used for the reconstruction, then the availability of tissue from other parts of the body (the back, for example) may be limited, and adding an implant can improve the breast form. The most common type is a latissimus dorsi flap.

Latissimus dorsi flap

This flap is formed from muscle and skin that is removed from the upper back with partial attachment and then tunneled underneath the skin from the back to the chest. Although this method provides much of the needed skin, there's usually not enough tissue to form the breast. Often the skin and muscle from the back will be stretched with either a tissue expander or implant. Then at a later stage, the tissue expander is exchanged with a permanent implant.

This type of breast reconstruction is commonly performed if you have had a mastectomy on one of your breasts and then radiation, if you don't meet the criteria for a TRAM or DIEP flap, or if you don't have enough excess abdominal tissue to form the breast. The latissimus dorsi flap isn't recommended if you perform strenuous or repetitious overhead arm activities.

Opposite breast balancing surgery (optional)

The best plastic surgeon still can't create a matching breast to your natural breast; there are always going to be variations. If you have large breasts, you may consider a breast reduction of the opposite breast to match the reconstructed breast. If your breast is small and has a sag, then you may need to lift your natural breast, augment, or add an implant to improve the shape and symmetry. All types of breast balancing procedures leave permanent scars on your breasts.

REMEMBER

If you're considering this option, your plastic surgeon will explain in detail the technique and the placement of the scars after the procedure.

Nipple-areola reconstruction (optional)

It is best for nipple reconstruction to occur after three to six months to allow your reconstructed breast to "settle" or for all the swelling to resolve. If you had radiation therapy, it's best for you to wait at least six months after completing radiation before reconstructing the nipple-areola. Waiting three to six months will allow the plastic surgeon to place the nipple and areola in the proper position. It will also allow the skin to heal after chemotherapy or radiation, which improves its ability to heal. Nipple-areola reconstruction is an outpatient surgery procedure with little discomfort.

The options for nipple-areola reconstruction include the following:

>> **Skin grafts:** Tissue from your abdominal scar from the DIEP/TRAM flap or inner crease of thigh or labial region (if you have undesirable excessive labial tissues) can be used as skin grafts for the nipple.

>> **Nipple sharing:** If you have a prominent nipple on your natural breast, a portion of it can be used as a skin graft to make a new nipple.

>> **Tattoo of nipple and areola:** A tattoo procedure is often done as a final process to match the color of your natural nipple and areola, either in a minor procedure room or by a medical tattoo artist several months following the nipple-areola reconstruction. Results can be quite good.

Nipple–areola reconstruction also allows the plastic surgeon to "nip and tuck" or make any adjustments that weren't done at the initial surgery, make any revisions such as removing "dog-ears" or extra skin from the mastectomy scar under the arm, or perform liposuction of the armpit.

EXTERNAL BREAST PROSTHESIS (BREAST FORMS)

Although this is not a surgical reconstruction option, it's a simple alternative if you don't want to have breast reconstruction surgery. There are many different types and styles of breast prostheses. The breast prosthesis may be built into a special bra or can be custom made to fit into a regular size bra. There are partial breast prostheses that are used to fill the space after a lumpectomy/partial mastectomy.

Advantages include the following:

- No risk from general anesthetic or surgery
- No extra scars
- Easy to use and take care of
- Satisfactory contour or shape in clothing

Disadvantages include the following:

- No natural tissue or reconstructed breast
- Need to hide under clothing and may slip out
- May limit the type of clothing you wear and may feel heavy or bulky
- May feel uncomfortable and hot in warm temperatures
- May cost several hundred dollars and sometimes is partially covered by insurance

Risks of nipple reconstruction include the following:

>> Bleeding

>> Infection

>> Poor wound healing

>> Loss of shape and height

>> Excessive flattening or shrinkage

>> Malposition of the new nipple

>> Skin graft failure

>> Additional scars on the reconstructed breast

There are a few alternatives to nipple–areola reconstruction:

>> Prosthetic nipple

>> 3D tattoo of nipple-areola

>> No surgery

Risks of Breast Reconstruction

There are always risks involved with any type of surgery, and breast reconstruction is no different. The plastic surgeon will discuss the risk of surgery at your clinic visit and will answer any questions you may have. Some of these risks include the following:

>> Bleeding, pain, scarring, and/or infection

>> Changes in sensation

>> Wound healing problems

>> Fluid buildup (such as hematomas and seromas)

>> Implant failure or disfigurement or loss of implants

>> Partial or complete loss of flaps

>> Abdominal hernia

>> Bulges

>> Asymmetry (lopsidedness)

>> Poor cosmetic results

Questions to Ask Your Plastic Surgeon

As always, don't hesitate to ask anything and everything you may be concerned about. Be sure to write questions down as you think of them — that way, you can bring the list to your pre-operative appointment or consultation. Examples include the following:

>> Will I be able to have breast reconstruction?

>> What types of reconstruction should I consider and which is best for me?

>> When can I have reconstruction done?

>> How many of these breast reconstruction procedures have you done?

>> Will the reconstructed breast match my remaining breast, and if not what can be done?

>> How will my reconstructed breast feel after surgery? Will I have any sensation?

>> What possible complications from the surgery should I know about?

>> How long will the surgery take? How long will I be in the hospital?

>> Will I need blood transfusions?

>> How long is the recovery time from surgery?

>> Would I need help at home to take care of my wounds?

>> How long after surgery can I start my exercise regimen or return to normal activity such as doing house cleaning, driving, and working?

>> May I talk to other women who have had the same surgery?

>> Will reconstruction cause a delay for chemotherapy or radiation therapy?

>> How long will the implant last? Do I have to replace it over time?

>> Is there any type of breast imaging (such as breast MRI) that should be done after implant?

>> What happens if I gain or lose weight? Do I have to change my implant?

Choosing Among Your Options

Breast reconstruction is considered an elective surgery and is intended to enhance your self-image and confidence after breast cancer surgery. If you're considering breast reconstruction, you should talk to the plastic surgeon about all options available to you. Only then can you make an informed decision.

The decision to have breast reconstruction is a personal one. There are physical and psychological benefits from breast reconstruction, but you must be committed to the process before you begin. If you're uncertain whether you want breast reconstruction, remember that you can always choose to undergo breast reconstruction later. The choice to have breast reconstruction requires careful and thoughtful consideration, and that decision is only yours to make. It is important that you discuss the breast reconstruction options with your plastic surgeon. Table 12-1 sums up some of the options.

TABLE 12-1   **Deciding between Implant/Expander or Autologous Tissue**

	Implant/Expander	Autologous Tissue
Surgery	Foreign object to create your breast mold	Your own tissue to create your breast mold
Hospitalization	Outpatient surgery or same-day surgery	Inpatient or in hospital surgery
Recovery	Shorter: 2 weeks after tissue expander placement	Longer: 6–8 weeks
Scars	Only mastectomy scar	Mastectomy scar plus scar from donor site
Shape and feel	Firm all over, no natural sag	Natural feel, soft

Note that Table 12-1 is just an average depiction of the process. Each patient is different and may have a different experience depending on other factors such as their medical history.

TIP

If you've completed breast reconstruction and aren't happy with the resulting shape or look, be aware that you can always have more surgery to improve things. No woman should have to live her life with a reconstructed breast that she's unhappy with. So let your plastic surgeon know how you feel. Sometimes getting the breast shape corrected requires more nipping and tucking.

If your plastic surgeon says that the fault or asymmetry of your breast can't be fixed, seek a second opinion. Some plastic surgeons are more skilled than others.

Chapter **13**

Treating Advanced Breast Cancer

The term *advanced breast cancer* may take on a different meaning, depending on the healthcare professional using the term. In this chapter, when we use the term *advanced breast cancer*, we're referring to breast cancers that can't be cured, also known as stage IV disease. Anytime a cancer can't be cured, that means it's more likely to grow, spread, and probably end your life. The question becomes: Will you die today, next year, or five or ten years from now — or longer? Your cancer doctor can give you an estimate of your life expectancy based on the stage of the disease and the organs involved. Your survival largely depends on the biology of your tumor (ER+ PR+ versus triple negative) and your health status. But you have some control (or input) over your disease, as your survival partially depends on the treatment and other factors that may be personal and important to you (including spiritual, emotional, natural, and other factors).

Advanced breast cancer (also called *secondary* breast cancer in the U.K.) means breast cancer that has spread to another part of the body, such as the liver, brain, or bones. Another term used to describe advanced breast cancer is *metastatic* breast cancer, or "incurable" cancer. Sometimes a patient is diagnosed with advanced breast cancer initially, and other times the diagnosis comes when breast cancer comes back (called *recurrent* breast cancer) after initial breast cancer treatment.

Even though there is no cure for advanced breast cancer, treatment can control it, relieve symptoms, improve your quality of life, and even prolong your life for a time.

Breast cancer typically spreads to the following locations (although it can eventually spread to any site):

>> Lymph nodes

>> Lung

>> Liver

>> Bones

>> Brain

If you or your loved one is diagnosed with advanced breast cancer, it is imperative that you listen to and understand what the doctor says about your treatment options.

Treatment Decisions and Treatment Options

In most cases, advanced breast cancer can be treated, and the goals of treatment must be clearly defined by your cancer doctor (medical oncologist). The goals of treatment for advanced breast cancer are often to relieve symptoms (palliation), shrink the cancer or slow its growth, and help you live longer.

There are people who are living longer with advanced breast cancer, in some cases five years, ten years, and more. Every person's cancer is unique, and your response to treatment may be different. Your cancer growth rate may also be different from the same type of breast cancer in someone else.

As advanced cancer grows, it can cause symptoms that may need to be treated to help control them. These symptoms can almost always be treated, even when the cancer itself is no longer responding to treatment.

Treatment decisions for advanced breast cancer

Treatments for advanced breast cancer are similar to treatments for early stage breast cancer. However, the differences are in the type of chemotherapy, endocrine therapy, and biological therapy and how long the treatment is given.

TIP

Making the decision about treatment can be difficult when you have advanced breast cancer. Although treatments with chemotherapy or radiotherapy can help relieve symptoms and might make you feel better, they also have side effects that can make you feel sick, though often the side effects are temporary. You have to go into treatment with "guns blazing" to have a fighting chance for a longer survival.

Here are four questions to ask your cancer doctor when making the decision for treatment:

» How will treatment benefit me? (Relieve pain and disease symptoms versus live longer or both?)

» How might treatment affect my quality of life?

» What are the side effects of treatment?

» How long will I need treatment?

Your cancer doctor or nurse can talk to you about the risks and benefits of treatment, as well as the side effects. It may be helpful for you to talk to a close friend, relative, or counselor about your treatment options to gain an objective outlook about your treatment decision.

Treatment options for advanced breast cancer

Your cancer doctor may consider the following before recommending a specific treatment for you:

» The size of the cancer and where it is in the body

» The types of treatment you have previously received

» Whether the cancer cells have receptors for particular types of drug treatment

» Your overall health status

» Your age

>> Whether you have had menopause

>> Whether the cancer is growing slowly or more quickly (how aggressive your cancer is)

>> Your genomic profiling

Genomic profiling is a laboratory method used to learn about the genes in a person and the way those genes interact with each other and with the environment. Genomic profiling may be used to find out why some people get certain diseases and others do not, or why people react in different ways to the same drug. It may also be used to help develop new ways to diagnose, treat, and prevent diseases such as cancer.

Advanced breast cancer may only respond to specific types of treatment, and your cancer doctor may start with the treatment that will give you the best results associated with the fewest side effects possible.

REMEMBER

Treatment can often keep advanced breast cancer under control for many months or even years.

The main types of treatment for advanced breast cancer include the following:

>> Endocrine (hormone) therapy

>> Chemotherapy

>> Radiation therapy

>> Biological therapy

>> Combination therapy (including endocrine, chemotherapy, and biological therapy in various groupings)

Endocrine or Hormone Therapy for Advanced Breast Cancer

Endocrine therapy is often called *hormonal therapy* and is a common treatment for advanced breast cancer (Chapter 11 talks a lot more about hormonal therapy). It can often reduce the size of the tumor and control the spread of the cancer wherever it is in the body. Endocrine therapy works well if the cancer cells have specific proteins called *hormone receptors*.

Our hormones are made naturally in the body and control the growth and activity of healthy normal cells. Prior to a woman reaching menopause, the ovaries produce the hormones estrogen and progesterone, and after menopause, body fat then produces estrogen. Most importantly, these hormones stimulate the growth of some breast cancer cells.

Endocrine therapy reduces the levels of estrogen and progesterone in the body, or blocks their effects on tissue. It can only work if the breast cancer cells have estrogen receptors (ER) or progesterone receptors (PR). Typically 70 percent of breast cancers have estrogen receptors (are ER+, meaning estrogen-positive). Your cancer doctor will check your cancer cells for estrogen receptors when you're diagnosed (no matter what stage of cancer you have).

Endocrine therapy is most beneficial for slow-growing breast cancers affecting the bones or the skin.

You might have endocrine therapy when your advanced breast cancer is first diagnosed, or after receiving chemotherapy treatment.

Here are the most common endocrine therapy medicines used for advanced breast cancer:

>> Anastrozole (Arimidex)

>> Exemestane (Aromasin)

>> Fulvestrant (Faslodex)

>> Goserelin (Zoladex)

>> Letrozole (Femara)

>> Medroxyprogesterone acetate (Provera)

>> Megestrol acetate (Megace)

>> Tamoxifen

More information on the length of therapy and side effects can be found in Chapter 11.

Chemotherapy for Advanced Breast Cancer

Your cancer doctor may suggest chemotherapy if your cancer doesn't have hormone receptors or has spread to the liver or lungs.

The goal of chemotherapy for advanced breast cancer is to relieve symptoms, control the cancer, and improve your quality of life for a time. Chemotherapy will not cure your breast cancer.

In many situations, the chemotherapy drugs for advanced breast cancer are the same as those used for early stage breast cancer. Your cancer doctor may consider the following factors before recommending a specific type of chemotherapy for you:

>> What chemotherapy drugs you've had before

>> How well the cancer responded to those drugs

>> What side effects you previously experienced from chemotherapy

>> Your overall health and fitness

Chemotherapy drugs that cancer doctors often use for advanced breast cancer include the following:

>> Docetaxel (Taxotere)

>> Vinorelbine (Navelbine)

>> Capecitabine (Xeloda)

>> Gemcitabine (Gemzar)

>> Paclitaxel (Taxol)

>> A type of paclitaxel called Abraxane

>> Epirubicin (Pharmorubicin)

>> Eribulin mesylate (Halaven)

Your cancer doctor may recommend one drug or a combination of drugs, to have the most benefit of relieving symptoms or controlling the cancer. For example, gemcitabine and paclitaxel, or capecitabine and docetaxel.

Chemotherapy is usually delivered directly into your bloodstream through an intravenous (IV) drip, whereas other chemotherapy drugs are given in tablets or capsules that you swallow. Chemotherapy treatment is given in cycles, such as every three weeks, and the patient will be reevaluated every three months to determine the treatment response. The side effects of chemotherapy are further discussed in Chapter 10.

Talk to your cancer doctor about your treatment plan, side effects from treatment, length of treatment, and when you should contact them about symptoms or side effects.

TIP

Biological Therapies for Advanced Breast Cancer

Biological therapies are drugs that change the way cells work and help the body control the growth of cancer. Biological therapies were created due to the immune system's failure to destroy faulty or damaged cells. Some biologics seek out and destroy cancer cells, whereas others help the immune system or body to attack the cancer. Chapter 11 talks more about biological therapies.

The immune system works to protect us against diseases, including cancer. It normally picks up faulty cells and destroys them, but sometimes the immune system misses these, and cancer develops. Scientists are working on ways to trigger the immune system so it can target cancer cells.

Biological therapy for advanced breast cancer can be given as any of the following:

>> An intravenous (IV) drip in your arm

>> An injection under the skin

>> A tablet

Role of HER2 receptors in advanced breast cancer

Two individuals can have breast cancer, but the type of breast cancer is different because of the presence or absence of biomarkers or proteins on the cancer cell.

Biomarkers can be proteins or receptors. They are measurable substances in the body found on the surface of breast cancer cells, within body tissues, and inside body fluids such as blood. *Human epidermal growth factor receptor - 2* (HER2) is a receptor made of protein that makes cells grow and divide. Some cancers have large amounts of HER2 protein and are called HER2–positive cancers, or HER2+.

Approximately 15–18 percent of newly diagnosed breast cancers have an abundance (or overexpression) of HER2 receptors which causes cancer cells to divide faster and survive longer. If you have HER2+ breast cancer, it means that your cancer is more aggressive, and that it can grow faster and spread quickly to other parts of your body. When HER2+ breast cancer spreads to other parts or *metastasizes*, the breast cancer is advanced.

Trastuzumab (Herceptin)

Trastuzumab goes under the brand name Herceptin and is a monoclonal antibody. A *monoclonal antibody* attaches to proteins on or in breast cancer cells. Herceptin targets and blocks the HER2 protein that stimulates breast cancer cells to grow and multiply. You can only receive treatment from trastuzumab if your breast cancer cells make too much of the protein.

Approximately 30 percent of people with advanced breast cancer have HER2+ breast cancer. The pathology from your breast biopsy will show whether your cancer is HER2+.

Trastuzumab can be given as an intravenous (IV) drip into your bloodstream or an injection under the skin (subcutaneous injection). Trastuzumab is usually given every 3 weeks for 12 months.

Trastuzumab may be given in the following ways:

» On its own

» With chemotherapy such as paclitaxel

» With hormonal or endocrine therapy

» With chemotherapy and another biological therapy (for example, pertuzumab)

» With other drugs as part of a clinical trial

Common side effects of trastuzumab include the following:

» Loose stools or diarrhea

» Irritation or redness at injection (IV) site

» Cold symptoms (stuffy nose, sinus pain, sore throat, sneezing)

» Stomach pain

» Belly or abdominal pain

- » Headaches
- » Joint or muscle pain
- » Back pain
- » Nausea/vomiting
- » Change in taste
- » Mouth sores
- » Loss of appetite
- » Insomnia or sleep problems
- » Fatigue or tiredness
- » Weight loss
- » Skin rash

Pertuzumab (Perjeta)

Pertuzumab also targets the HER2 protein, but it blocks a different part of the protein than trastuzumab.

Pertuzumab is sold under the brand name Perjeta and is a monoclonal antibody. Pertuzumab works by attaching onto HER2 in the cancer cells to stop their growth and eventually kills them. Pertuzumab only works if your cancer is HER2+.

Pertuzumab can be given as an intravenous (IV) drip into your bloodstream. Your first treatment will take over 60 minutes as your team checks you for any side effects. Subsequent treatments take between 30 and 60 minutes. You will be given pertuzumab every three weeks.

You can have the infusion through a thin short tube (a *cannula*) that goes into a vein in your arm or you can have it through a central line, a PICC (peripherally inserted central catheter) line, or a port-a-cath — long plastic tubes that deliver the drug into a large vein in your chest. The tube stays in place throughout the course of treatment.

Most people may experience one or more of the following side effects:

- » Breathlessness and looking pale
- » Bruising more easily
- » Constipation

>> Diarrhea

>> Feeling or being sick

>> Hair loss

>> Increased risk of getting an infection

>> Loss of appetite

>> Nausea

>> Pain

>> Skin changes

>> Sore mouth

>> Tiredness and weakness

REMEMBER

Tell your doctor or nurse if you have any side effects so they can help you manage them. Your nurse will give you a contact number to call if you have any questions or problems. If in doubt, call them.

Denosumab (Prolia, Xgeva)

Denosumab is another type of monoclonal antibody. When cancer spreads to the bones, it can cause your bones to become weak and painful.

In healthy bones, specialized cells constantly break down and replace old tissue. This process is called *bone remodeling* and is very well controlled. These specialized cells are of two types:

>> Osteoclasts break down old bone.

>> Osteoblasts build new bone.

There is a narrow balance between the rates of bone breakdown and growth, which keeps bones strong and healthy. Denosumab works by targeting a protein called RANKL, which controls the activity of osteoclasts. This stops bone cells being broken down and strengthens the bone. Denosumab can strengthen the bones to lower the risk of fractures and help to control pain.

Denosumab is given as an injection just under your skin (subcutaneously). How often you have Denosumab depends on the brand. Xgeva is given once every four weeks. Prolia is given every six months.

Common side effects of denosumab include the following:

>> Nausea

>> Fatigue

>> Muscle weakness

>> Low levels of phosphorus in the blood (hypophosphatemia)

Less common side effects of denosumab include the following:

>> Shortness of breath

>> Cough

>> Headaches

>> Eczema (skin condition that may include redness of the skin, itching, dryness, swelling, blistering, or bleeding)

>> Back pain

>> Joint pain

>> Limb pain

>> Skin rash

REMEMBER

Most people will not experience all the side effects listed for denosumab. The side effects are predictable in terms of onset, duration, and severity and are likely to improve after treatment is completed. Denosumab side effects are very manageable and there are several options available to minimize or prevent the side effects.

Everolimus (Afinitor)

Everolimus goes under the brand name Afinitor. It's a biological therapy that is used for a few types of cancer, including advanced breast cancer. Everolimus is given when you have been through menopause (you're postmenopausal) and in combination with the endocrine therapy medicine exemestane.

Everolimus is a signal transduction inhibitor that stops some of the signals within cells that make them grow and divide. Everolimus stops a particular protein called mTOR from working normally and stops the cancer cell from growing or slows down the growth.

Everolimus is given as a tablet once a day. You should take everolimus at the same time each day and swallow it with at least 8 ounces of water. You can take it with or without food. But you must take it the same way every day — with food or every day without food. If you miss a dose, don't take an extra dose. Take the next prescribed dose at the usual time. You usually take everolimus every day for as long as it works.

Common side effects of everolimus include the following:

>> Anemia (low red blood cell count)

>> Mouth sores

>> Infection

>> Weakness/fatigue

>> Cough

>> Increased creatinine

>> Diarrhea

>> High cholesterol level

>> High triglyceride level

Less common side effects include the following:

>> Nausea/vomiting

>> Shortness of breath

>> Lung problems

>> Poor appetite

>> Elevated liver enzymes

>> Swelling or generalized edema

>> Fever

>> Nosebleeds

>> Fatigue

>> Low blood counts (white blood cells and platelets; white blood cells are part of the immune system and responsible for fighting off infection)

>> Itching

>> Dry skin

Other issues with biological treatment

You'll have blood tests before starting treatment and during your treatment. The team checks your levels of blood cells and other substances in the blood. They also check how well your liver and kidneys are working.

Immunizations

Don't have immunizations with live vaccines (rubella, mumps, measles, yellow fever, or Zostavax or shingles vaccine) while you're having treatment and for at least six months afterwards.

You can do the following:

>> Have other vaccines, but they might not give you as much protection as usual

>> Have the influenza vaccine

>> Be in contact with other people who've had live vaccines as injections

You must do the following:

>> Avoid contact with people who've had live vaccines taken by mouth (oral vaccines). This includes the rotavirus vaccine given to babies. The virus is in the baby's urine for up to two weeks and can make you ill. So, avoid changing the diapers for two weeks after their vaccination.

>> Avoid anyone who has had oral polio or typhoid vaccination recently.

Pregnancy and contraception

Don't become pregnant or father a child while you are having chemotherapy treatment with these drugs and for at least six months afterwards. This drug can harm the unborn child. Your doctor may advise you not to take the contraceptive pill because the hormones in the pill may affect your breast cancer. Talk to your doctor or nurse about effective contraception before starting treatment.

Little is known about whether or not chemotherapy medicines can pass through vaginal secretions or semen. Therefore, as a precaution, your doctor may advise you to use a barrier method (such as condoms or femidoms) during vaginal, anal, or oral sex. Generally, doctors advise a barrier method only for the time you are actually having the treatment and for about a week after your treatment.

Advice like this can be worrying, but it doesn't mean you have to avoid being intimate with your partner. You can still have close contact with your partner and continue to enjoy sex.

Treatment for other conditions

Always tell other doctors, nurses, or dentists that you're having biological treatment if you need treatment for anything else, including teeth problems.

Blood clots

You are more at risk of developing a blood clot during treatment. Drink plenty of fluids and keep moving to help prevent clots.

Breastfeeding

Don't breastfeed during treatment because the drug may come through in your breast milk.

Other medicines, foods and drink

WARNING

Cancer drugs can interact with other medicines and herbal products. Tell your doctor or pharmacist about any medicines you are taking. This includes vitamins, herbal supplements, and certain over-the-counter remedies. Some of these supplements and herbs to avoid while receiving chemotherapy include the following:

» **Acidophilus:** May cause infections or other problems if taken during chemotherapy.

» **Astragalus:** May interfere with certain immunosuppressants.

» **Coenzyme Q10, selenium, vitamins A, C, and E:** The antioxidant properties may interfere with the effectiveness of chemotherapy because they help to prevent cell damage and may stop the chemotherapy from working well.

» **Echinacea**

» **Fish oil:** May increase bleeding.

» **Ginger:** May increase bleeding.

» **Green tea:** May reduce benefits of certain anticancer drugs.

» **Licorice:** May affect estrogen levels.

» **Milk thistle:** May affect estrogen levels, which could pose an issue for breast or ovarian cancer.

>> **Reishi mushroom:** May interfere with certain drugs or chemotherapy.

>> **St. John's wort:** May cause increased bleeding.

>> **Turmeric:** May reduce the effectiveness of chemotherapy — or increase the effects, with toxic results.

Radiation Therapy for Advanced Breast Cancer

Radiation therapy can shrink breast cancer tumors, relieve symptoms, and help you feel more comfortable (see Chapter 9 for much more about radiation therapy). You can have radiotherapy to different areas of the body at the same time.

Radiation therapy can treat breast cancer that has spread to the following areas:

>> One or more areas of bone

>> The skin

>> The lymph nodes

>> Parts of the brain

Radiation as injection

If your breast cancer can spread into several places in the bone, you may be offered strontium 89 (also called by its brand name, Metastron). This type of radiation will help to control the pain.

Strontium 89 is given as an injection into a vein. It circulates through your body and is taken up by the cancer cells in the bone. The amount of radiation from the injection is small and does not cause any harm to anything else. But it can kill cancer cells.

Side effects of radiation for advanced breast cancer

Radiation side effects typically start a few days after the radiation begins and worsen as treatment continues and can continue to get worse after your treatment ends. But side effects usually begin to improve after one or two weeks. Everyone is different and may or may not experience certain side effects.

Side effects can include the following:

» Tiredness and weakness

» Feeling or being sick

» Reddening or darkening of your skin

» Loss of hair in treatment area

Tell your cancer doctor or nurse about the radiation symptoms you experience and for how long, so they can be managed with medications.

End of Life Concerns

End of life discussions are usually initiated when the provider or the cancer team has determined from your medical status and disease state that you have six months or less to live. It is difficult for your doctor to give an accurate prediction of your life expectancy after a diagnosis of advanced breast cancer because more and more people are living longer due to the innovations in chemotherapy and biological therapies.

Advanced stage breast cancer is often treated as a chronic disease, like diabetes and hypertension, because it may not affect your day-to-day life and there are treatments that can be given if a medical problem arises. However, for some life can be more challenging with having to receive constant treatment (chemotherapy, biological therapy, and endocrine therapy) in order to control the spread of the disease and its symptoms.

Whatever your circumstances, you'll need to come to terms with the fact that you may not live as long as you might want to live. You may be constantly thinking about whether you have weeks, months, or years left to live and what death will be like.

The thought of dying sometimes can be more frightening than death itself because it is perceived in terms of loss of control and dignity. If you understand how well your symptoms can be effectively controlled and the available support system throughout your care, your fear me be reduced, and you can focus on living well for the remainder of your days on earth.

Receiving psychosocial support is important. That may come in the form of counseling, education on your disease, financial counseling, or spiritual services such as going to church. Getting support for coping with your disease and treatment is a key facet to helping you live well and maintain a positive outlook on life.

Communicating to Providers

You and your providers should have a close patient-provider relationship, so you can share with them the symptoms you're having and they can help you manage them. You are an integral part of the effective management of your symptoms. Your cancer doctor won't know what you are experiencing at home if you do not call them and let them know. Besides your cancer doctor liaising with your team, they are often reaching out to your primary care doctor or general practitioner to ensure that your care is integrated.

Tell your cancer doctor if your breast cancer or treatment interfere with your ability to

>> Be social or engage in recreational activities.

>> Think clearly.

>> Sleep.

>> Maintain relationships with family and friends or participate in family life.

>> Work (have lost income or difficulties with disability insurance).

>> Have intimacy or sexual relations with partner.

>> Be emotionally healthy.

>> Be physically active (exercise, play sports) or function in other ways.

When you openly share your concerns and partner with your healthcare team, you're more likely to receive quality care because

>> You feel more in control.

>> Your treatment will be more in alignment with your preferences, needs, and goals.

>> You get greater patient satisfaction and buy-in for complying with your treatment plan.

>> Your diagnosis is less frightening.

4

Dealing with Breast Cancer and Everyday Life

Be knowledgeable about psychosocial concerns when it comes to breast cancer diagnoses.

Get help in managing the stress that often comes with diagnosis and treatment.

Find out how to better cope with changes that occur after treatment.

Check out tips on maintaining your sexuality and fertility despite breast cancer.

Make healthy lifestyle changes to improve your well-being.

Chapter **14**

Psychosocial Concerns and Breast Cancer Diagnosis

Although breast cancer is one of the most common cancers among women, it is highly treatable and even curable if it is diagnosed in the early stages (stage I or II). At this time there are more than 3.1 million breast cancer survivors in the United States. This includes women still being treated and those who have completed treatment. As we have mentioned a few times, breast cancer is often treatable and even curable in the early stages. Breast cancer is *not* a death sentence. Medical research, technology, and current treatment options are much better than what was available 20 years ago.

REMEMBER After treatment and recovery, many breast cancer survivors lead full, productive, purposeful, healthy lives. However, some breast cancer survivors experience difficulties in their life post cancer. There is a variety of resources targeted to providing supportive care to breast cancer survivors.

Some cancer survivors and their loved ones or close supporters are at risk for a number of health-related distresses — including depression, sadness, anxiety/panic, fear, worry, or anger — as a result of the breast cancer diagnosis and treatment effects. Distress is usually expected in the immediate stage of breast cancer diagnosis and treatment. However, some of the negative side effects and emotional challenges can linger long after the completion of treatment. Your sense of self and identity, and parts of your life like work, family, social life, relationships, and intimacy, may be affected.

Fear and Worry and Their Physical and Emotional Toll

Psychological health is important for cancer survivors and is defined by the presence or absence of distress and worry as well as the presence or absence of positive emotional growth and physical well-being. Your psychological health is determined from the balancing of worry/distress and the support and resources available to cope with the stress or burden.

The physical impact of breast cancer and its treatment varies on the extent of the cancer, the treatments, the survivor, and their living and social situation. The stage at which the cancer is diagnosed usually determines what type of treatments you will receive and how long it will last. Some common early physical changes due to all the treatments include tiredness/fatigue, pain, vaginal problems, weight gain, and menopausal symptoms. These physical problems are more common among women who receive chemotherapy and hormonal therapies. However, these more intensive and whole body system treatments can save lives. The physical discomforts, plus the distress of adjusting to cancer, may have a negative effect on a woman's emotional, social, and spiritual well-being. Research shows that women of Latin and African descent report greater physical and functional (work and daily living) challenges. However, most of these symptoms decrease over time and are often gone within two years, especially if the survivor receives good follow-up medical and supportive care.

For some survivors, the physical changes resulting from cancer treatment come with emotional distress as well. You may experience depression — feeling very sad and having a deep sense of loss.

Concern for children being at a higher risk for cancer, the recurrence of cancer, and even fear of death are common. As a result, both depression and anxiety are common among cancer survivors.

Almost everyone who's had breast cancer worries about whether the cancer will come back. Almost every ache, pain, rash, or lump can frighten you, but as time goes by you will get to know your "new normal," which may include symptoms that just occur because you have had breast cancer treatment. You may find you experience frequent stressful events, such as the days leading up to your first mammogram after breast cancer treatment, or labs, especially if you just got news that someone you knew got a recurrence of breast cancer or even died. Cancer can create feelings of anxiety or constant worry among some survivors. In addition, *scan anxiety* is often manifested while survivors are waiting for the results from MRI, PET, or CT scan, or even labs.

Fear of cancer recurrence is associated with the following:

>> Poorer quality of life and greater distress

>> Lack of planning for the future

>> Avoidance of, or excessive follow-up

>> Greater health care utilization

>> Effect on mood and relationships

Depression and anxiety are two of the natural, though unhealthy, ways that our bodies respond to extreme stress, and that includes dealing with cancer. Research conducted to examine the impact of cancer on quality of life and cancer outcomes among survivors revealed that Latina and Korean Americans reported the poorest emotional and psychosocial well-being. For most survivors, the depression and anxiety will decrease gradually over time. However, for a few survivors depression is a troubling emotion that continues and leads to the following:

>> Desire to get away from everything

>> Difficulty enjoying things

>> Disturbed sleep patterns

>> Fatigue

>> Feeling hopeless about the future

>> Irritability

>> Physical symptoms (such as pain)

>> Uncontrollable crying

Anxiety is another troubling emotion that can continue and lead to the following:

>> Being easily distracted

>> Depression

>> Feeling dizzy, drowsy, and tired

>> Feeling irritable, impatient

>> Heart palpitations, racing heart

>> Muscle aches

>> Nausea/sick to stomach

>> Trouble focusing

>> Trouble sleeping

>> Restless

You may also have repeating thoughts that affect your daily life, cause difficulty breathing, or affect your ability to relax.

Later in this chapter we offer suggestions to help you cope with depression and anxiety.

Women who feel that the ability to have children is an important part of being a woman often suffer a greater sense of loss when radiation and/or chemotherapy treatments prevent them from having children. This sense of loss can affect intimate and family relationships. (See Chapter 17 for more on sexuality and intimacy.) Survivors may experience the loss of their breasts as a loss of their womanhood or femininity. Due to the cancer and its treatments, they may see themselves as less desirable. A woman may also be fearful about losing the partner or spouse who cannot adjust to the new changes in her body. Later in this chapter we offer helpful strategies to help you cope with body image and intimacy concerns.

Functional Concerns: Work and Home Life

After breast cancer treatment you may experience changes in your physical functioning or experience a feeling of disability when you're unable to complete activities such as cooking, housekeeping, or laundry, or even to care for yourself and family.

Cancer can change how you relate to people in your life. Cancer can bring you and your family and friends closer. However, cancer and its treatments can create distress due to pain, fatigue, lymphedema (swelling), losing your hair, as well as a sense of loss. These changes to your health, appearance, and emotional state may cause you to avoid family and social activities.

Research shows that survivors have expressed concerns about disclosing their illness and burdening their families (Ashing-Giwa et al., 2003, 2004, 2006). Specifically, Asian and Latina Americans reported inadequate familial coping and support, Chinese Americans reported the use of positive coping activities, while Korean Americans endured more negative feelings among their family. These concerns often decrease over time as you adjust to your new body. Changes may also occur in your intimate relationship, resulting in changes in your roles. For example, your partner may want to do more caretaking. Adjusting to cancer can cause hurt in some relationships, yet many relationships are strengthened by the cancer experience. Cancer can even result in new friendships through support groups and getting involved in community organizations. Later in the chapter we provide information and a variety of resources to help you maintain or regain a sense of confidence regarding each of these issues.

Functional capability for occupational activities

Occupational activities are often taken for granted but are related to the human needs of self-care, entertainment, and social participation. Occupational activities are often engaged in based on cultural norms, values, and beliefs so that structure can be maintained in an individual's life. The following are the seven major domains of occupational activities:

>> Basic activities of daily life

>> Instrumental activities of daily life

>> Play

>> Sleeping and resting

>> Leisure

>> Formal education

>> Social participation

In addition to occupational activities, functional capability must be understood because it is associated with your ability to perform certain basic activities independently. Because functional capability is focused on your ability to perform a task, it's linked to the preservation of motor-muscle strength and cognitive skills that relate to quality of life.

Some cancer survivors complain of changes in memory, or "chemo brain," which can involve difficulty in coordinating activities or multitasking, and difficulty raising hands above the head, which are functional changes with occupational activities. Physical and occupational rehabilitation is known to be effective in reconditioning your muscles by improving motor skills as well as occupational activities.

WARNING

If you have developed any of these cognitive or physical changes, you should let your doctor know so you can be referred to rehabilitation.

Fear of infertility

One significant after-effect of cancer treatment is infertility, where a premenopausal woman is unable to get pregnant because of limited or no ovarian function.

Studies have shown that minorities and individuals of African descent are more likely to experience infertility, even if they don't have cancer treatment. Researchers reviewed differences in rates of infertility and utilization of infertility services in the United States in three selected areas of reproductive health: infertility, polycystic ovary syndrome (PCOS), and reproductive aging. Results of this study showed that in addition to having higher rates of infertility, women of African descent presenting for infertility care have a longer duration of infertility compared with Caucasian women. In addition, among minorities, Asian women in Massachusetts — where there is a higher education and income level compared with other racial and ethnic groups — had a higher rate of infertility treatment compared to their Caucasian counterparts or African counterparts in that population. These findings suggest that differential access to care is based on either economic or sociocultural barriers. When you consider the shortened fertility period that occurs from the side effects of chemotherapy and radiation, *oncofertility* services (the field that focuses on the reproductive capabilities of cancer survivors) become more urgent for those desiring future fertility after a diagnosis of cancer.

Questions have been raised concerning the estrogenic effects of medications used to increase fertility after cancer treatment on women with a history of estrogen-based cancers. For example, a doctor shouldn't give clomifene (sold as Clomid, an estrogen receptor modulator frequently used for infertility) to a woman with a history of an estrogen-receptor-positive breast cancer because estrogen is the very hormone you would like them not to take. The better process is to preserve fertility prior to treatment.

Ask your doctor about preserving your fertility before starting cancer treatment. If fertility is important to you, then make it a priority. It's not acceptable for a doctor to tell you that seeing a fertility specialist will delay your cancer treatment. Eggs or ova can be harvested within two weeks of treatment.

If you didn't get the opportunity to preserve your fertility prior to treatment, it's not too late to talk to a fertility specialist. Both the fertility specialist and your oncologist should discuss the best fertility options that are available for you.

Worrying about work and finances

The cost of treatment for cancer often can change your financial situation for a variety of reasons. Women with cancer are often faced with medical bills that are higher than expected. A cancer diagnosis may cause changes to your insurance coverage, including cost increases, and may even result in your being dropped from your insurance altogether. There are policies or safeguards in place currently in the United States to prevent loss of insurance from pre-existing conditions, but these may not last forever, and this may not be true for other places around the world. You may lose work time in order to attend medical appointments or to recuperate from treatments.

For women who work outside the home, a diagnosis of cancer may affect the ability to keep the job you already have or to find a new one. A diagnosis of cancer can create concerns about job security, promotion, and your ability to perform well at work.

You don't have to let anyone know about your cancer diagnosis unless you feel it's necessary to tell them. You may choose to tell your employer if you're physically unable to do your job responsibilities. For example, sometimes surgery to the abdominal area, lymphedema (discussed in Chapter 16), or "chemo brain" can affect your ability to lift things and do physically active jobs. Although you may feel as though your health challenges are private issues, in some cases, it may help to communicate with supervisors and co-workers at your place of employment.

The following are suggestions to help you discuss important issues with supervisors and co-workers:

>> If your employer knows about your cancer diagnosis, you may want to inform them that you intend to perform your best at work.

>> If you need to work part-time for a while until your strength and energy return, ask if this is a possibility. You can talk to the personnel manager to see whether working part-time would affect your benefits and insurance status.

>> You can ask your doctor to write a letter explaining your health status. This may also be helpful as documentation if your employer needs to excuse you for routine and follow-up appointments.

>> If you're unable to do your old job due to physical limitations, you can ask your employer about working in a different department or giving you less physically demanding work.

Spirituality

Cognitive spiritual coping is beneficial to getting through the physical and emotional burden of breast cancer treatment and recovery. Cognitive spiritual coping occurs in the following 11 dimensions:

>> **Relinquishing control:** Giving up your desire for control to a higher power or your spiritual meaning system

>> **Social comparison:** Comparing your breast cancer experiences to others for cognitive relief of your distress

>> **Trauma recall:** Remembering the crises moments during breast cancer diagnosis and treatment and recounting how your spiritual beliefs helped you to cope with the stressor

>> **Idealized spiritual attribution:** Viewing the negative events in your life as a positive experience that a higher power has allowed for your purposeful growth

>> **Universal interconnectedness:** Embracing advocacy, philanthropy, and other activities that can benefit others

>> **Prayer/meditation:** Engaging in prayer for yourself or others, as well as in relaxation techniques and mindfulness

>> **Spiritual services:** Attending church, Bible studies, prayer groups, mass, and so on

>> **Spiritual texts:** Reading the Bible, daily devotionals, memoirs, self-help books, and so forth

>> **Gratefulness:** Self-reflecting and having feelings of gratitude for your breast cancer journey

>> **Peace:** Sense of satisfaction, calm, and comfort that helps you to cope well with cancer through your focus on spirituality and meaning

>> **Transcendent awareness:** Feeling connected to God, a higher power, nature, self, or others

Seeking Support

Like many, you probably have different roles to handle in everyday life. Perhaps you are a daughter who is caring for an elderly parent. You may be a mother, wife, employee, and volunteer. Many single women are the primary breadwinners and nurturers of families. Others have probably come to rely upon your abilities to do many things well. So how will the world continue to revolve when you are sick? Better yet, who will care for you?

These are the questions women with breast cancer ask themselves. Moreover, no matter how well you communicate with family members, no one, other than someone who has experienced it, can truly understand the discomfort, fear, and uncertainty that a cancer diagnosis brings. Some women find that a support group can offer the comfort and support that they need to endure treatments and beat cancer.

Purpose and benefits of participating in a support group

Support groups allow people who are experiencing similar situations to share their concerns and problem-solving strategies. Newly diagnosed members may find it helpful to hear how other women deal with the medical system, how they communicate with their children, and about how they cope with the uncertainty of the illness. Additionally, support groups can provide information, education, support, and advocacy. Extra support may be especially helpful to single, divorced, separated, and widowed women, who may not have children or extended family that they can rely on for help. Support groups provide emotional support and may provide transportation assistance, escorts to treatment, and other resources. Having another person with the same religious, spiritual, or cultural beliefs with you can be comforting and reduce some of the stress that comes with cancer and its treatments.

How support groups are structured and organized

Support groups can vary in structure and function. They may be run by professionals (for example, oncologists, social workers, psychologists, psychiatrists, oncology nurses, or clergy) or by cancer survivors. Groups may be open, allowing group members and their families to come and go for as long as the group is running. Closed groups are more structured, beginning and ending with the same members for a specific period. Group meetings may have planned topics that are discussed, or group meetings may have a free-flowing format, allowing members to express whatever their experiences and concerns may be that day. The sites where groups meet can also vary. Meetings may be held in intimate settings such as a person's home, or in churches, educational sites, hospitals, or community agencies.

After you've found the type of group that is right for you, it may take some time to become comfortable enough to share your experiences. Different people have varying comfort levels for talking about their feelings or about their health concerns and family issues. Know that your discomfort is normal and that in time, with the support and understanding of those around you, you will be able to share with the group.

How to find a support group

There are many local, regional, and international support groups or support networks for breast cancer survivors. Collectively support groups' main goal is to provide emotional, physical, or financial support by providing resources to assist the breast cancer survivor throughout treatment and beyond. Support groups can be organized at the grassroots level, where a cancer survivor or a community advocate wants to help or give back, and other times it may be formed out of a health or religious organization and even local or state governments. The key is knowing how to find the breast cancer support group or network that will best fit your needs.

TIP

Appendix B lists several of the most popular breast cancer organizations and networks. Check it out for more information on support groups and other resources.

> » **Knowing the importance of sleep and how to improve it**

> » **Getting to know complementary therapies such as acupuncture and meditation**

> » **Checking out how to manage depression and anxiety and seeking support and professional care**

Chapter **15**

Managing Stress

Stress is a normal part of life. But besides the stresses of daily life such as paying bills and managing a career and family, women who have a serious illness like cancer have the added stress of coping with the disease and its treatments. In addition, for persons with the cancer diagnosis, there is the fear that the cancer may return, fear of disease progression, fear of treatment side effects, and fear of death.

When we feel extreme stress, it may be experienced as a symptom of depression and anxiety. The following are symptoms of depression, and these symptoms are common among cancer survivors:

>> Difficulty coping

>> Feelings of helplessness or hopelessness

>> Difficulty focusing on tasks and concentration

>> Memory problems

>> Changes in appetite (overeating or undereating)

>> Changes in sleep habits (insomnia, oversleeping, or staying in bed all day)

>> Lethargic with no energy

>> No fun or interest in activities that used to be enjoyable

>> Frequent tearfulness and sadness

>> Feeling isolated and alone

Symptoms of anxiety can include the following:

>> Feeling nervous, restless, or tense

>> Having a sense of impending danger, panic, or doom

>> Having an increased heart rate

>> Breathing rapidly (hyperventilation)

>> Sweating

>> Trembling

>> Feeling weak or tired

>> Trouble concentrating or thinking about anything other than the present worry

>> Having trouble sleeping

>> Experiencing gastrointestinal (GI) problems

>> Having difficulty controlling worry

>> Having the urge to avoid things that trigger anxiety

WARNING

If you have these symptoms for more than two to four weeks, talk to your doctor about a referral for counseling and therapy. Your therapist may also refer you for an evaluation for a brief course of medication to help relieve the symptoms.

No cancer survivor should feel that they have failed or feel ashamed because of feeling depressed and anxious. Cancer is a very traumatic experience, and periods of feeling distressed, depressed, and anxious are common.

TIP

Medications to relieve the depression and anxiety are helpful for cancer survivors. Medications may take 15 days or several weeks to work. The most common side effects experienced in the first two weeks are nausea, headache, and dry mouth.

Sertraline, citalopram, and escitalopram have the fewest drug-drug interactions and are well tolerated. Antidepressant selection can also be guided by the dual benefit that several of these medications may improve not only depression but also cancer-related symptoms such as anorexia, insomnia, fatigue, neuropathic pain, and hot flashes.

TIP

Many breast cancer survivors find it helpful to speak with a counselor, support group, or minister to share their concerns and receive support for their problems during initial and ongoing treatment. Even one visit to a qualified counselor/therapist can make a difference.

Many cancer survivors experience ongoing fears of cancer recurrence, and this chronic uncertainty of health status during and after cancer treatment can be a significant psychological burden. Some patients who experience severe distress may require psychological and pharmacological interventions such as therapy or antidepressants, respectively. Your emotional well-being deserves top priority for your physical and psychological health, so you should be concerned more about self-maintenance of health and not overly worry about the unknown.

REMEMBER

Depression and anxiety are common emotional reactions to cancer diagnosis and treatment. Seeking group support can help manage depression and anxiety among cancer patients. Other strategies to manage depression and anxiety include mindfulness-meditation, massage, acupuncture, yoga, problem-solving therapy, and cognitive behavioral therapy. You can talk to a family member or seek the help of a professional if the depression and anxiety are too overwhelming. In such instances, you can call the CRISIS hotline at 800-784-2433.

REMEMBER

Seeking help is not a sign of weakness — it's a sign of *strength*.

BE ACTIVE AND HAVE SOME FUN

A mounting set of new research shows evidence that healthy eating and fun, physical activity provide effective stress relief and reduce symptoms of depression and anxiety. Light to moderate body movements for about 30 minutes at least four to five times a week — such as walking, dancing, and exercise — can offer symptom relief and a feeling of well-being and improve mood and joy. Healthy eating with a plant-based diet and limiting animal-based foods to no more than two times a week (if you eat meat) are highly recommended. There is growing evidence of clear physical benefits to healthful eating and regular fun body movements, including having more energy, enjoying better and more restful sleep, and reducing the risk of cancer recurrence.

For cancer patients, finding a licensed therapist can be very rewarding for both the patient and family. Many doctors will encourage their patients and caregivers to seek a therapist. Counseling can provide support and guidance for patients to explore ways to manage any emotional concerns. Family counseling can be beneficial for helping the patient's family to learn different ways in coping with their emotions that may result from caring for their loved ones. Sometimes the patient and family just need someone to talk to, to help them work through their experience with cancer. These counseling sessions are healthy and productive ways to release stress and reduce anxiety that may result during and after treatment. Oncology social workers also help patients and family better understand the healthcare system and options for treatment and life after cancer.

Incorporating Relaxation Techniques

Many people with cancer find that practicing deep relaxation relieves their pain and stress. At first, these relaxation exercises can feel unfamiliar, and everyone needs time and practice to see them work. Relaxation helps our positive thoughts and energy flow more easily through our bodies.

You can practice relaxation in a comfortable chair or even on your bed. If you choose a chair, be sure to keep your legs uncrossed. If you find that you're rushing it, slow yourself down and remember that part of feeling relaxed is to slow down your thoughts and breathing. Once you find a comfortable spot, you can begin.

REMEMBER

It's important to remember not to do any exercise that feels painful or uncomfortable. Start slow and easy.

Go through the following script, saying the words to yourself in a calm, easy manner.

I will learn to relax my muscles. As I focus on each part of my body, I will tighten my muscles and hold the tension for ten seconds and then release quickly. All the while I am tensing and releasing my muscles, I will focus on my breathing. By breathing slowly and deeply, I will fill my lungs as much as I can, and then let all the air out very, very slowly. I will be asked to tense (squeeze) each of my muscle groups for ten seconds and then relax completely. I must use my diaphragm (the muscle under my ribs) to breathe deeply. As I release all the tension from my muscles, I'll feel the difference when they are relaxed.

1. Beginning with my body, I will tighten and relax the muscles in my feet and toes.

2. I am tightening and releasing my ankles and shins. Taking my time, I will give each part of my body some attention. I can focus on different areas of my body for a few seconds or for a few minutes . . . now, my knees and thighs.

3. I am tightening and relaxing my buttocks, where I feel the most pressure if I am sitting in a chair. I notice if the muscles in my buttocks are tense, and if they are, I will relieve the tension and relax the muscles. As I get rid of the tension in my muscles, I am letting feelings of peacefulness move through me.

4. Next, I tighten and relax my stomach and chest area. I notice whether I feel tension in my chest area. I will take a few deep gentle breaths and slowly release them. I am letting go of all the tension that I've been holding in this area. I will take a slow and steady breath.

5. Now I tighten and relax my shoulders and my neck. I will take my time focusing on this area. We tend to hold a lot of stress here. As I focus on my shoulders and my neck, I will take a deep, slow breath and release all the tension that I have been holding here. I will take another deep, gentle breath and slowly release.

6. I am tightening and relaxing my forearms and my hands. I am letting my fingers relax, and I am taking a deep and gentle breath.

7. Next, I tighten and relax my neck and my face. I let my head and neck relax. I notice if I am tense in this area. I breathe slowly and deeply and slowly release.

8. Now I am tightening and relaxing my mouth and tongue.

9. At last, I can relax my eyes and let them sink. Ahhh . . . I take eight slow, deep, healing breaths. I notice how good it feels to be totally relaxed.

After practicing tensing and relaxing, you can do the relaxing without the tensing. With time and patience, you can soothe your body and mind by doing the following:

>> Always finding a quiet time and place where you can rest undisturbed for 20 minutes

>> Letting others know you need this time for yourself

>> Making sure your setting is relaxing

Your relaxing setting can be achieved by doing the following:

>> Dimming the lights and finding a comfortable chair or couch

>> Getting into a comfortable position where you can relax your muscles

>> Closing your eyes and clearing your mind of distractions

>> Breathing deeply at a slow and relaxing pace

>> Raising your stomach rather than just your chest with each breath

Visualization exercise: Lying in a meadow

I will create a relaxing place in my mind:

>> I imagine that it is a calm and peaceful summer day, and I am out in a meadow.

>> I have a soft, cotton blanket that I spread on the smooth ground, and I'm lying on that blanket.

>> The sun is off to one side, so I can comfortably look up at the blue sky and the clouds.

>> I can feel the warmth of the sun on my face and shoulders and can see the long grasses around me moving slightly in the gentlest of breezes.

>> I hear the gentle sound of birds singing, echoing faintly, and the scent of the trees.

>> I watch the clouds moving slowly overhead. I notice the edges of the clouds. They contrast with the blue sky.

>> I feel the calm and peace all around me and within me.

>> Now, that scene slowly drifts away — and I let it go.

>> I come back to the feelings of pure relaxation.

>> I notice where I feel most relaxed, how my mind may have slowed down. Perhaps I'm drifting or feel some other sensation associated with relaxing.

>> I will enjoy this feeling of relaxation.

>> As I breathe out, I will let any remaining bits of tension drift out of my body.

TIP

The first time you go to your relaxing place, you may stay for two or three minutes. You can stay longer if you like, nurturing your body, mind, and healing spirit.

The Importance of Sleep

Sleep is vitally important to our health and well-being. Sleep helps to replenish energy for the body and mind to be able to problem-solve and concentrate in our daily lives.

To help you get a better night's rest, try the following tips:

» Avoid eating a heavy meal or drinking a lot of liquids (tea, soda, water) close to bedtime to avoid waking up to use the restroom.

» Keep a regular sleep schedule, including weekends. Say goodnight and arise at consistent times. If you get enough sleep, you'll wake up on your own. Avoid caffeine, alcohol, and nicotine —and remember, drinks such as most sodas, hot chocolate, tea, and coffee are high in caffeine. They work as stimulants, they're addictive, and they keep you awake.

» Exercise in the early part of the day to improve mood, energy, and well-being. Exercise also increases your ability to get deep, refreshing sleep. And it decreases fatigue and helps you stay healthy. You should avoid exercising two to four hours before bedtime to give your body an opportunity to calm down and prepare for sleep.

» Keep your sleeping environment cool. Metabolism naturally slows at night, and the quicker you can relax, the better. Cooling seems to slow people down both physiologically and mentally. You can use an air conditioner or fan to keep the room cool. Instead of keeping the furnace on high during the winter, layer your pajamas and add more blankets to your bed to keep you comfortable.

» Sleep only at nighttime and go to bed only if you're sleepy. Limit any daytime sleep to brief naps.

» Keep it quiet. Turn off the radio and TV. If necessary, a constant, soothing sound such as from a fan or white noise machine in the background will help cover up undesirable noise.

» Make your bed and make sure your bed and mattress are supportive and comfortable. If you wash and change bedding every week, you'll have a healthier sleeping environment.

» Relax — practice the relaxation exercise in the previous section.

» Beware of sleeping pills. Check with your doctor before using them. It's important to make sure the pills won't interact with other medications or with an existing medical condition. Never mix alcohol and sleeping pills. If you feel sleepy or dizzy during the day, talk to your doctor about changing the dosage or stopping the pills.

» If you're having trouble sleeping, use your bed only for sleeping and intimacy. Avoid reading, watching TV, or eating in bed.

» If you can't fall asleep after 30 minutes, get up and go into another room. Try doing something else and then return to bed when you're ready to go to sleep. If you return to bed and are again unable to sleep, get up and leave the room again. This helps connect your mind to your bed as a signal for sleep.

TIP

Consider taking a hot bath or shower before bedtime to help put you in a nice tranquil state before dozing off.

Spirituality and Meditation

Studies have shown that spirituality often serves an essential part of one's healing after cancer. Although feeling the initial fear upon hearing the cancer diagnosis is natural, spirituality can provide a source of comfort, support, emotional stability, meaning, and purpose. Many African American and Latina American survivors in our studies said that their spirituality sustained them during the treatments and in their life after cancer. They emphasized the significance of prayer, faith, and their spiritual community in coping with and recovering from cancer.

Some survivors initially see their cancer diagnosis as a spiritual challenge. This "questioning of faith" is a very common experience after a cancer diagnosis. Others see the cancer as a calling to become more spiritual.

Many cancer survivors report that cancer causes them to view life in a new light and re-evaluate what they value most. Cancer can set a new agenda for life and can propel the survivor to greater heights. Some survivors have described it as attaining mental stability, finding your true self, undergoing a spiritual awakening, or making reconnection. Whereas some women have described their faith and spirituality as providing sustenance and bringing meaning to their lives, others expressed mixed feelings and difficulty making sense out of their experience. However, many survivors find support through their faith or religious community and comfort in gathering with people who have similar experiences.

REMEMBER

Most survivors are able to draw strength from their spirituality and find higher peace and purpose through the cancer experience.

Tips for finding comfort, meaning, and spiritual support

The following are some ways to help achieve a feeling of spiritual meaning during your cancer experience:

>> Find faith-based support by contacting religious or spiritual leaders in your community.

>> At your place of worship, ask for resources such as counseling and support groups for people with chronic illnesses like cancer.

>> Join a faith-based support group where you can share and hear others' experience and spiritual journey after cancer.

>> Join a prayer group to pray and share your fears and concerns.

>> Read religious or spiritual books and articles that bring meaning and focus to life.

>> Ask your hospital, healthcare providers, or social worker about faith-based organizations that provide specialized services for survivors.

>> Visit religious gatherings to meet new people, especially those who have a similar life experience.

>> Seek spiritual guidance from within as well as from people in your spiritual or religious community on how to use the cancer for a greater purpose.

>> Help others who have had cancer through volunteering with your spiritual community, hospital, or organizations like the American Cancer Society, Wellness Community, and Susan G. Komen Foundation.

>> Join a research study to benefit both yourself and others.

Many people who are diagnosed with cancer experience a need to become closer to their spiritual and religious beliefs. The following visualization exercise can be helpful in connecting with your spirituality. Please keep in mind that this is only a guide. You can use and adapt the following as affirmations, prayers, and/or meditation in any way you choose. You can add to these affirmations as you please. For example, you can add words from prayer or worship or as the spirit moves you.

Call for inner peace

Using contemplation and spirituality can provide stress relief for some:

>> Lead me from spiritual isolation into your presence.

>> Lead me from worry into inner peace.

>> Lead me from fear into power.

>> Lead me from family discord/conflict into family unity.

>> Lead me from stress into harmony.

>> Lead me from social isolation into the nurturance of companions.

>> Lead me from pain into comfort.

>> Lead me from sadness into joy.

>> Lead me from doubt into purpose.

>> Lead me from sickness into health.

>> Lead me from patient into survivor into victor.

This section by Dr. Kimlin Tam Ashing originally appeared in "Embracing Hope: Hopeful Living After Breast Cancer."

Health affirmation

Try this affirmation for health-related stress. This can be used as a meditation or recited as an affirmation for wellness:

>> My body is a temple: strong and resilient.

>> I am protected and covered by the divine one.

>> I feel the warmth of healing light.

>> My whole body is washed in healing waters.

>> My immune system and bodily defenses against illnesses are plentiful.

>> My immune system is perfectly tuned to detect and remove any cancer cells.

>> With each breath, I am closer to wellness.

>> With each breath, I am closer to wholeness.

>> With each breath, I am closer to harmony.

>> I am nourished and calm, yet powerful and protected.

This section by Dr. Kimlin Tam Ashing originally appeared in "Embracing Hope: Hopeful Living After Breast Cancer."

ACUPUNCTURE

Complementary and alternative medicines, also called CAM, are becoming more common among cancer patients and cancer survivors. Acupuncture, a traditional Chinese medicine that has been used in the United States for about 200 years, involves needles in different places on the skin called *acupuncture points*. It is used to treat many illnesses and pain in cancer patients and may help relieve symptoms such as nausea and vomiting, fatigue, neuropathy, anxiety, and depression. Acupuncture treatment should be given by a qualified practitioner.

Chapter **16**

Coping with Changes after Treatment

Cancer treatment can save lives, but those lives then often undergo many changes — some expected, others unexpected. This chapter aims to cover many of these changes and offer advice on dealing with them constructively.

TIP

No survivor should have to face cancer alone. Seek out people among your family and friends who can participate in your doctor visits, help keep track of your medical symptoms and records, and help you get the best medical care and resources. See Appendix B for suggestions on resources.

Cancer-Related Fatigue

Fatigue is a familiar experience in daily life. It means you have little or no energy to perform work, enjoy activities, or focus on important matters. Usually all you need is about eight hours of sleep and your fatigue will be history — you'll be re-energized and fully functional in your cognitive abilities.

Unfortunately, cancer-related fatigue is much worse than regular fatigue. It's the kind of fatigue that doesn't resolve with sleep and it causes significant distress. It's a feeling of being drained, "washed out," and weak. You may be too tired even to walk to the bathroom, take a shower, or eat. You may have difficulty thinking or processing thoughts or in moving your body from side to side. This type of fatigue causes even more distress when symptoms of depression, pain, nausea, or vomiting are manifested. Cancer-related fatigue can last a long time, is unpredictable and overwhelming, and it affects your quality of life. It also affects your caregivers' quality of life because they will have to do more to support you during this period.

Recognizing cancer-related fatigue

The American Cancer Society has compiled the following signs of cancer-related fatigue:

>> You feel tired and it doesn't get better — it keeps coming back or it becomes severe.

>> You're more tired than usual during or after an activity.

>> You're feeling tired and it's not related to any activity.

>> You put less energy into your personal appearance.

>> You're too tired to do the things you normally do.

>> Your arms and legs feel heavy and hard to move.

>> You have no energy and feel weak.

>> Your tiredness doesn't get better with rest or sleep.

>> You spend more time in bed and/or sleep more, or you have trouble sleeping.

>> You stay in bed for more than 24 hours.

>> You become confused.

>> You can't concentrate or focus your thoughts.

>> You have trouble remembering things.

>> Your tiredness disrupts your work, social life, or daily routine.

>> You feel sad, depressed, or irritable.

>> You feel frustrated and upset about the fatigue and its effects on your life.

Managing cancer-related fatigue

Here are some tips for managing cancer-related fatigue:

>> Improve your sleep time and incorporate a routine of activities where you listen to soothing music or read before bedtime. Avoid intake of caffeine, alcohol, and tobacco after mid-afternoon because they can keep you awake.

>> Develop a routine for your other daily activities. You may find that you have more energy in the morning, so plan important activities around the times when you have the most energy.

>> Take short naps and rest periodically during the day. Plan your naps around the times when you are most fatigued. Rest often before you feel tired.

>> Try to avoid activities that make you feel more fatigued. You may have to seek help from friends or family to help complete the important activities that you may not be able to do. This may also be the time to talk to a social worker or nonprofit organizations that may be able to help with transportation, cooking, cleaning, and so on.

>> Make your preferences known to friends and family. Some people undergoing treatment prefer not to talk on the telephone because they find conversation exhausting. If you feel this way, ask friends to drop you a note or send a text or email instead of calling. Many people use an answering machine or voicemail to screen their calls when they are fatigued. That way you can talk to people when you feel up to it. Others find that talking with loved ones is helpful. In this case, tell people how much their calls mean to you and ask them to call often.

>> Talk to your doctor or nurse for help with things that add to your fatigue such as pain, nausea, and sleep problems. There are medications that can help you manage those symptoms and reduce your fatigue.

>> Follow a healthy diet by eating small, well-balanced, high-protein meals and snacks throughout the day. Less energy is required to digest small meals than larger meals. Talk to your doctor or nurse about whether there is any benefit from taking vitamins during this period. Your nutritionist can also help with this.

>> Be socially active and don't cut yourself off from your friends. Spending time with friends, family, and church members is important, but you must remember to pace yourself.

- » Walk daily. Light exercise increases blood circulation and your energy level.

- » Get emotional support. Your family, friends, and religious organizations can help you deal with stress and fatigue. You may also want to join a support group for people with cancer.

- » If you have anxiety and depression, ask your doctor or nurse for help. Learning yoga, mindfulness, acupuncture, and other relaxation techniques can be helpful.

- » Activities of daily living can be improved with the help of an occupational therapist (OT). The OT is skilled in helping you perform essential activities without getting you fatigued. Talk to your doctor or nurse to see whether an OT is right for you.

Dealing with Hair Loss

This is the one we're all familiar with from TV shows and movies. Most chemotherapies will result in hair loss all over the body and head. Radiation therapy can also cause hair loss in the area being treated. Some endocrine therapies, such as those involving letrozole, also can lead to partial or complete hair loss. You should definitely talk with your healthcare team regarding your treatment to see if it will lead to hair loss.

TECHNICAL STUFF

This hair loss is technically known as *alopecia*.

There are several ways to manage the hair loss caused by chemotherapy and radiation therapy:

- » **Treat your hair gently.** You may want to use a hairbrush with soft bristles or a wide-tooth comb. Don't use hair dryers, irons, or products such as gels or clips that may hurt your scalp. Wash your hair with a mild shampoo, wash it less often, and be very gentle. Pat it dry with a soft towel.

- » **Know you have choices.** Some people choose to cut their hair short to make it easier to deal with when it starts to fall out. Others choose to shave their head. If you choose to shave your head, use an electric shaver so you won't cut yourself. If you plan to buy a wig, get one while you still have hair so you can match it to the color of your hair. If you find wigs to be itchy and hot, try wearing a comfortable scarf or turban.

- » **Protect and care for your scalp.** Use sunscreen or wear a hat when you're outside. Choose a comfortable scarf or hat that you enjoy and that keeps your head warm. If your scalp itches or feels tender, using lotions and conditioners can help it feel better.

>> **Talk through your feelings.** Many feel angry, depressed, or embarrassed about hair loss. It can help to share these feelings. Some find it helpful to talk with others who have also lost their hair during cancer treatment. Talking with your children and close family members can also help you all. Tell them you expect to lose your hair during treatment.

Caring for your hair when it begins to grow back

Hair loss isn't usually permanent. Take good care of it when it starts to regrow:

>> **Be gentle.** When your hair starts to grow back, you will want to be gentle with it. Avoid too much brushing, curling, and blow-drying. You may not want to wash your hair as frequently as you used to before cancer.

>> **Care for it after chemotherapy.** Hair often grows back within two to three months after treatment. Your hair will be very fine when it grows back. It may be curlier or straighter — or even a different color — than before. In time, it may go back to how it was before treatment.

>> **Care for it after radiation therapy.** Hair often grows back within six months after treatment. Unfortunately, with a very high dose of radiation, it may grow back thinner or not at all on the part of your body that received radiation.

>> **Hydrate on the inside and outside.** Drink lots of water and add fruit or spices like fresh ginger or basil to help make it more interesting. Hydrate hair on the outside by conditioning after washing or washing using only conditioner, and by adding water when you brush it.

Talking with your healthcare team about hair loss

Prepare for your visit by making a list of questions to ask in advance. Consider adding the following questions to your list:

>> Is treatment likely to cause my hair to fall out?

>> How should I protect and care for my head? Are there products that you recommend? Ones I should avoid?

>> Where can I get a wig or hairpiece?

>> What support groups could I meet with that might help?

>> When will my hair grow back and what will it look like when it does?

Addressing Skin Changes

Sometimes changes to the skin occur as a result of cancer treatment. This section talks about some ways to address these changes.

Understanding discoloration and hyperpigmentation

Your skin may change color at various stages of breast cancer treatment. The most common skin change is called *hyperpigmentation*, or darkening of the skin. The following are the causes of skin discoloration:

>> **Surgery:** scarring post-surgery can make the skin darker or lighter.

>> **Radiation:** During radiation treatment, you may notice the color of your skin, from pink to red. If you're of African descent or have a dark brown or black skin tone, the redness is difficult to see but you may still have dryness and soreness of the skin.

>> **Chemotherapy:** During intravenous chemotherapy treatment you may notice your skin and veins becoming darker or discolored. The skin changes can be widespread or only at or around a specific area on your body. Skin color changes are more common in areas of the skin that are exposed to the sun and in darker-skinned individuals.

>> **Injection site reaction:** During the injection of some chemotherapy or other treatment medications a site reaction may occur with tenderness, warmth, redness, or discoloration along the vein closest to the injection site. This is called *vesicant extravasation*. Vesicants cause blistering and severe skin damage that may be severe and lead to tissue death. Chemical cellulitis is caused by some of the contents of the injection not getting into the vein and leaking out under the skin or in the tissue.

>> **Skin rash:** During certain chemotherapy treatments a rash or recall can develop before or after receiving radiation.

The following are some of the more common areas that are often affected by discoloration. Areas that may become blotchy include the following:

>> Along the vein used to infuse chemotherapy

>> Around the joints

>> In the hair (horizontal bands in light-haired individuals)

>> In the mouth

>> Under areas compressed by tape or dressings

>> Under the nails

There are two main types of cancer treatment–caused discoloration:

>> **Radiation discoloration:** The deep redness and the sensitivity should start to go away during the first weeks after radiation. Your skin will take longer to return to its natural color. Sometimes the treated area will be darker or have a tan for up to six months after your last radiation treatment.

>> **Chemotherapy discoloration:** Symptoms of discoloration typically occur two to three weeks after chemotherapy treatment begins. These symptoms begin to go away as new skin cells replace the dead cells, at approximately 10–12 weeks after treatment is over.

REMEMBER

Discoloration of the skin from cancer treatment can sometimes be permanent or take a longer time to resolve. In other words, the darkening may occasionally be permanent.

Experiencing Numbness and Tingling: Peripheral Neuropathy

Numbness and tingling in the hands and feet are known as *peripheral neuropathy*, and the sensations are caused from damage to the nerves. Chemotherapy can cause nerve damage, especially medicines such as vinca alkaloids (vincristine), cisplatin, oxaliplatin, paclitaxel, and the podophyllotoxins (etoposide and tenoposide). Other drugs used to treat cancer, such as interferon and thalidomide, can also cause nerve damage.

Being at increased risk for peripheral neuropathy

Individuals who are at greatest risk for developing peripheral neuropathy after chemotherapy are (but aren't limited to) those with pre-existing conditions that can cause nerve injury. These conditions include the following:

>> Alcoholism

>> Diabetes

>> Previous chemotherapy

>> Severe malnutrition

TIP

The symptoms of the nerve damage caused from certain chemotherapy medicines are exactly the symptoms that can develop when a person's diabetes or blood glucose is not controlled.

Unfortunately, glucose control will not help chemo-induced peripheral neuropathy. High glucose levels in the blood and chemo damage nerves by different cellular mechanisms, but result in similar clinical presentations. Sometimes this is described as a "glove and stocking" pattern, as it develops in small nerves at the end of the hands and feet. Some of the medications that help control the symptoms of diabetic nerve pain can also be used for chemo-induced neuropathy, but they don't reverse the process and can have side effects.

Knowing the symptoms of peripheral neuropathy

The following are the most typical symptoms associated with peripheral neuropathy:

>> Burning sensation in hands and/or feet

>> Constipation

>> Difficulty picking things up or buttoning clothes

>> Loss of positional sense (knowing where a body part is without looking)

>> Loss of sensation to touch

>> Numbness around mouth

>> Numbness, tingling (feeling of pins and needles) in hands and/or feet

>> Weakness and leg cramping or any pain in hands and/or feet

The areas mostly affected by neuropathy include the following:

>> **Bowels:** The condition may cause or worsen constipation and may lead to conditions such as *ileus* (a paralysis of the bowels). Normally the bowels are contracting to move content all the time. An ileus can lead to blockage, but technically you do not have a full blockage if you have an ileus.

>> **Fingers and toes:** This is the most common version. The numbness will move gradually upward in a stocking-glove type fashion.

>> **Other places:** Sometimes the face, back, and chest are affected.

Signs of neuropathy mostly develop gradually and can worsen with each additional dose of chemotherapy. It is usually strongest right after a chemo treatment and tends to lessen just before the next treatment. The symptoms usually reach a peak about three to five months after the last dose of chemotherapy and thereafter may disappear completely, or lessen only partially. They may also merely affect less of the body.

If neuropathy is resolving, then it's likely to be a gradual process, usually requiring several months. However, in some cases it may be irreversible and never diminish in intensity or size of the area of the body affected.

REMEMBER

It's important to let your cancer team know when the symptoms of neuropathy are getting worse so they can adjust the dose of chemotherapy or perhaps end the treatment to avoid permanent nerve injury. Don't keep your neuropathy to yourself.

Reducing the effects of neuropathy from chemotherapy

There is no one-size-fits-all solution, sorry to say. But there are several techniques that you can use to prevent or reduce the severity of peripheral neuropathy from chemotherapy. Most of the treatment is based on trial and error and figuring out what works best for you.

Be sure to do the following:

>> Report any unusual feeling you may have to your healthcare professionals. Let them know if you are experiencing any of the symptoms described earlier so they can assess.

>> Follow instructions given to you regarding rest and delays in treatment.

>> Be active in decisions regarding following treatment versus maintaining your quality of life.

Try the following to increase your protection against peripheral neuropathy:

>> Protect areas of your body that feel numb or where sensation is decreased. For example, don't walk around without footwear. Rather, wear thick socks and soft-soled shoes.

>> Avoid exposure to extreme temperature changes, which may worsen symptoms.

>> Wear warm clothing in cold weather. Protect feet and hands from extreme cold.

>> Be careful when washing dishes or taking a bath or shower. Don't let the water get too hot.

>> Use potholders when cooking.

>> Use gloves when washing dishes and gardening.

>> Inspect your skin for cuts, abrasions, and burns every day. Be especially vigilant in checking arms, legs, toes, and fingers.

The following are tried-and-true comfort measures you can take to partially alleviate the symptoms:

>> Massage the area.

>> Use flexible splints to support joints.

>> Apply lotions and creams to keep the skin moist.

Relieving constipation induced by neuropathy

Try the following in order to lessen any constipation you may be experiencing:

>> Eat foods high in fiber like fruits (such as pears and prunes), cereals, and vegetables.

>> Drink two to three liters of nonalcoholic fluids (such as water and juices) each day — unless you're told otherwise by your doctor.

>> Exercise 30 minutes most days of the week, as tolerated, and after checking with your doctor to see if exercise is okay. A lot of patients find that walking for exercise is convenient and easy to do.

>> If you've been prescribed a "bowel regimen" that includes a fiber supplement, laxative, or increasing water intake to be taken at specific times throughout the day, make sure you follow it exactly.

Also, if you're taking narcotic painkillers (opioids), it will increase your risk of developing constipation. Conservative use of opioids can help significantly with constipation. Using alternative pain medication (such as NSAIDS, Tylenol, Motrin, topical pain relievers, warm or cold compress, and so forth) is often recommended for patients with chronic to severe constipation as approved by their healthcare provider.

TIP

Some patients have found deep breathing, relaxation, and guided imagery particularly helpful to reduce pain associated with neuropathy. See Chapter 15 for more on these techniques.

Checking out medications and treatments prescribed for neuropathy

Your oncologist may interrupt your chemotherapy treatment or reduce the dose to prevent worsening of this side effect. In addition, the oncologist may take any of the following actions:

>> Recommend that you use vitamins from the B-complex family (such as vitamins B-6 and B-12).

>> Control neuropathic pain by prescribing any of the following:

- Pain reliever (analgesic)

- Antidepressant (such as amitriptyline)

- Anti-seizure medication (such as gabapentin)

>> Recommend physical therapy. This may help with strengthening of muscles that are weak. Usual exercises include range of motion, stretching, and massage. Assistive devices such as orthotic braces, canes, and appropriate splints may also be recommended.

>> Recommend occupational therapy. This will help with assistive devices for activities of daily living. Therapies such as biofeedback, acupuncture, or transcutaneous nerve stimulation (TENS) may also be recommended/ prescribed in severe cases.

» Notify your other healthcare professionals if you're experiencing any of the preceding symptoms.

» Note unrelieved pain despite use of pain medications.

» Note constipation despite laxative use.

Coping with Lymphedema

The removal of lymph nodes under the arm, or injury can cause swelling under the arm or in the arm on the same side where the lymph nodes were removed. This condition is called lymphedema. *Lymphedema* occurs when areas of the body become swollen due to an increased amount of lymphatic fluid that can't drain.

In the case of breast cancer, the most common cause of lymphedema is the removal of the lymph nodes (not a decrease in lymph node function). Once the lymph nodes are removed, the associated lymphatic channels that drain the arm and normally empty into those lymph nodes in the arm pit are backed up. The fluid in the lymphatic channels then seeps out of the channels and into the tissue (that is, in the arm or underarm). Lymphatic fluid is clear to milky white fluid that is made up of the extra fluid that is produced in all normal tissues. One of the jobs of the lymphatic system (in addition to immune function) is to drain the extra fluid that normally accumulates in the healthy tissue.

After removal of the lymph nodes, mastectomy, lumpectomy, or radiation treatment, some women may experience a decrease in lymph node function in their underarm area, resulting in lymphedema.

There is a difference in risk of developing lymphedema of the arm with an SLNB (sentinel lymph node biopsy, where one to three lymph nodes are removed) versus a complete axillary dissection/lymphadenectomy (where all the lymph nodes are removed). It is a big difference: 0–5 percent risk of lymphedema after an SLNB compared to 20–25 percent after axillary dissection. A few decades ago, women were routinely getting axillary dissections, which is why there were so many lymphedema cases. Now fewer women are getting axillary dissections, and there is much less lymphedema.

Many women are often unsure whether they can do things like get an IV or blood pressure measurement in their arm after an SLNB. Once women with an SLNB have completely healed after surgery (6–12 months) and have no signs of lymphedema, it is generally okay to use that arm. For women with an axillary dissection, they should never use their arm for IV access, blood pressure readings, or any arm procedures.

The lymphatic system is responsible for fighting infection and disease in the body. More specifically, the lymph nodes contain lymphocytes and other cells that activate the immune system and filter substances that can be harmful to the body.

Lymphedema may occur within a few days of surgery and be mild and short-term. But it may also occur weeks, months, or years after the initial treatment has ended. Sometimes lymphedema can become long-term and increase the risk for infection. It's important to know the symptoms of lymphedema and to seek medical attention immediately if symptoms arise.

Knowing the symptoms of lymphedema

The following are the major symptoms:

>> Feelings of tightness in the arms, swelling of the arm

>> Rings feeling too tight on the fingers

>> Weakness in the arms

>> Pain, aching, or heaviness in the arms

Treatment for lymphedema

If you develop or suspect that you have lymphedema, you should see your surgeon or breast nurse as soon as possible.

Treatment for lymphedema is focused on reducing the swelling in the arm and preventing the fluid from building up again. Treatment has to be consistent because it takes some time to see results. Treatment may consist of any of the following:

>> Wear a compression elastic sleeve on your arm, from the wrist to the top of your arm near your armpit.

>> A compression elastic glove may be required to reduce the swelling in your fingers.

>> Wear a compression elastic vest to reduce breast or chest swelling.

>> The lymphedema specialist or therapist may use a special type of stretch bandage to wrap your arm to manage the swelling.

>> You may receive a manual lymphatic drainage (MLD), which is a special type of massage technique.

>> Your lymphedema specialist or therapist may teach you special exercises to help drain the fluid in the arm.

>> Your lymphedema specialist or therapist may order a compression pump to help divert the fluid from your arm to other areas of the body. You can read more about one of the types of compression pumps that is commonly used to manage lymphedema at www.tactilesystems.com.

>> During your clinic or treatment visits your lymphedema therapist, physical therapist, or breast nurse may measure your arm and request information about your symptoms.

TIP

The most beneficial way to manage lymphedema is to do the recommended exercises at home and to wear your compression sleeve when you are doing exercises, cooking, gardening, or any other activities that involve the dominant use of the affected arm.

WARNING

Stop exercising if your affected arm becomes red, warm, and sweaty. This may be a sign of poor lymphatic drainage and result in increased fluid accumulation at the site that eventually can lead to pain, discomfort, and physical limitation of the arm.

Taking preventative measures

As frequently as possible, keep your arms elevated above your heart. Clean the skin of your arms daily and moisturize with lotion. You may avoid injury or infection by doing the following:

>> Using an electric razor when shaving

>> Wearing gardening and cooking gloves

>> Using thimbles for sewing

>> Not cutting cuticles around your fingernails

>> Avoiding sun tanning and use sunscreen with at least 50 SPF or above

>> Cleaning and disinfecting cuts with soap and antibacterial ointment

>> Using gauze wrapping instead of tape, and wrapping loosely to avoid cutting off circulation

>> Talking to your doctor about any rashes

>> Avoiding needle sticks in the affected arm

>> Avoiding extreme temperatures or use of ice/heat packs

- » Not using blood pressure cuffs on the affected arm

- » Not wearing tight clothing with tight elastic bands

- » Not carrying a purse on the affected arm

- » Watching for signs of infection such as redness, pain, swelling, or fever and calling a doctor if any of these symptoms appear

- » Doing exercises regularly as prescribed by your doctor

- » Keeping regular follow-up appointments with your doctor

- » Checking extremities for symptoms on a daily basis

- » Eating a healthy diet

- » Avoiding becoming overweight

- » Learning as much as you can about the condition

Resources for lymphedema management

The following resources can provide you with more information about lymphedema:

- » **Lymphedema Resources, Inc.:** The organization's website is at www.lymphedemaresources.org.

- » **National Lymphedema Network Marilyn Westbrook Fund:** This is for patients who don't have insurance or the financial means to purchase the much-needed compression stocking(s)/sleeve(s). Check out www.lymphnet.org.

- » **Lymphedivas:** This site provides medically correct fashion for lymphedema sufferers. Check out www.lymphedivas.com.

- » **Lymph Notes:** There is an online lymphedema support group at www.lymphnotes.com.

- » **National Rehab:** This company sells compression pumps. Call 1-800-451-6510. They have locations in western and central Pennsylvania, eastern Ohio, and northern and eastern West Virginia.

- » **Flexitouch system:** Call 866–435–3948 or visit www.tactilesystems.com.

- » **Fitness and exercise advice for patients with lymphedema:** Check out www.lymphnet.org/pdfDocs/nlnexercise.pdf.

DEALING WITH PAIN

Cancer, treatment for cancer, and diagnostic tests can all cause pain. Each patient needs their own personal plan to manage cancer pain. Talk to your healthcare team about pain control. They may be able to help improve your quality of life during and after cancer treatment and diagnostic testing.

Changing Tastes and Smells

Cancer treatments can change your senses of taste and smell, and that in turn can affect your appetite (see next section). You may experience a bitter or metallic taste in your mouth. If you're having problems like these, try the following:

» Try new foods, marinades, spices, drinks, and ways of preparing foods that are different from your usual preparation.

» Keep your mouth clean by rinsing and brushing, which may help foods taste better.

» Avoid using silverware and instead use plastic utensils, cups, and plates.

» Use fresh or frozen fruits and vegetables instead of canned.

» Eat natural or sugar-free mints, gums, or hard candy.

» Try seasoned foods with lemon, ginger, citrus fruits, or vinegar. (But you should avoid citrus if you've developed mouth sores.)

» Try pickled foods.

» Flavor foods with spices such as garlic, onion, cilantro, basil, oregano, tarragon, parsley, rosemary, mint, cayenne pepper, pimento, ketchup, mustard, and more.

» You can counter a salty taste with added sweeteners, a sweet taste with added lemon juice and salt, and a bitter taste with added sweeteners.

» Rinse your mouth with a baking soda, salt, and water mouthwash before eating to help foods taste better. (Mix 1 teaspoon salt and 1 teaspoon baking soda in 1 quart water. Shake well before swishing and spitting.)

» Serve foods cold or at room temperature. When foods are hot, the heat can increase the smells and tastes of flavors you may not be able to tolerate.

» Freeze fruits like mango, strawberry, pineapple, cantaloupe, grapes, oranges, and watermelon. Then eat them as frozen treats.

» If red meats taste strange, try other protein-rich foods like chicken, fish, eggs, or cheese.

>> Make smoothies or frozen drinks by blending fresh fruits with milk, ice cream, or yogurt.

>> To reduce smells, cover beverages and drink through a straw.

>> Choose foods that don't need to be cooked.

>> Avoid eating in rooms that are stuffy or too warm.

Countering Changes in Appetite

It will be difficult for you or your doctor to predict how your breast cancer treatment will affect your appetite. There are times when you may continue to eat and enjoy your favorite meals, and there are other times when you don't feel like eating — or want to eat everything in sight. The changes in smell and taste (see preceding section) do affect appetite. It's best to be flexible and try new foods and new meal times as your body's needs change.

Appetite changes can be caused by almost all breast cancer treatments:

>> Surgery

>> Chemotherapy:

- Capecitabine (Xeloda)

- Carboplatin (Paraplatin)

- Cyclophosphamide (Cytoxan)

- Daunorubicin (Cerubidine, DaunoXome)

- Doxorubicin (Doxil, Adriamycin)

- Epirubicin (Ellence)

- Ixabepilone (Ixempra)

- Methotrexate (Amethopterin, Mexate, Folex)

- Mitoxantrone (Novantrone)

- Thiotepa (Thioplex)

>> Endocrine/hormonal therapy:

- Anastrozole (Arimidex)

- Exemestane (Aromasin)

- Fulvestrant (Faslodex)
- Letrozole (Femara)
- Nolvadex (Tamoxifen)
- Raloxifene (Evista)
- Toremifene (Fareston)

» Radiation therapy

» Targeted therapy:
- Bevacizumab (Avastin)
- Everolimus (Afinitor)
- Palbociclib (Ibrance)

» Lapatanib (Tykerb)
- Trastuzumab (Herceptin)

» Pain medication:
- Acetaminophen and codeine
- Fentanyl (Actiq, Duragesic, Fentora)
- Hydrocodone (Hysingla ER, Zohydro ER)
- Hydrocodone/acetaminophen (Lorcet, Lortab, Norco, Vicodin)
- Hydromorphone (Dilaudid, Exalgo)
- Meperidine (Demerol)
- Methadone (Dolophine, Methadose)
- Morphine (Astramorph, Avinza, Kadian, MS Contin, Ora-Morph SR)
- Oxycodone (OxyContin, Oxecta, Roxicodone)
- Oxycodone and acetaminophen (Percocet, Endocet, Roxicet)
- Oxycodone and naloxone (Targiniq ER)

TIP

If you have loss of appetite, here are some suggestions for improving it:

» Eat small amounts of high-protein and high-calorie foods every two or three hours instead of three large meals a day. High-protein foods include meat, fish, eggs, dairy foods, beans, and pulses.

» Eat puddings and desserts — foods with fat or sugar are good sources of calories.

» Try having family members or friends prepare your food. Cooking your own food can sometimes put you off eating.

» Add extra calories and protein to any food that you eat (using butter, milk, cream, sugar, honey, and cheese).

» Choose foods that have great aromas so that they appeal to your sense of smell.

» Prepare and store small servings of your favorite foods ahead of time so there is always something to eat when you feel hungry.

» Have a stock of convenient foods in the cupboard such as canned soups and puddings.

» Don't be afraid to try out new foods and tastes — you may be surprised at what you like.

» Chew food well and eat slowly.

» Don't give yourself a hard time if you really don't feel like eating for a few days after treatment. It's important to drink fluids, but you can make up for lost calories between treatments.

» Avoid getting overly tired — you'll find everything more difficult to cope with if you're exhausted.

» Avoid filling your stomach with a large amount of liquid before eating. Drink after your meal.

TIP

If you're worried about losing weight, ask your doctor about high-calorie meal replacement drinks.

Dealing with weight gain

Weight gain is quite common during and after breast cancer treatment. Women typically gain 5–15 pounds during treatment, and the more weight you gain, the less likely you are to return to your weight pre-breast cancer treatment.

Chemotherapy can cause you to gain weight in the following ways:

» Steroids given during chemotherapy can cause your body to hold excess fluid and increase your appetite.

» It may trigger craving for specific foods that may be high in fat and sodium.

» Chemotherapy by itself can cause your body to hold excess fluid.

» Fatigue causes inactivity, thus increasing weight gain.

» You engage in less physical activity, often because of fatigue.

>> Nausea is improved by increased eating.

>> Your metabolism slows down, along with your ability to burn fat and produce energy.

>> It may induce premature menopause in some women, which reduces metabolism.

REMEMBER

Steroid medications are given during breast cancer treatment for the following reasons:

>> To treat nausea

>> As part of the treatment for the cancer

>> To reduce inflammation, swelling, and pain

Managing weight gain

The causes of weight gain can vary. This is why you should talk to your doctor or nutritionist before attempting to adopt a specific weight loss diet or a change in your eating habits.

Basic proven methods for weight loss include the following:

>> Eat plenty of fruits, multicolored vegetables, and whole grains.

>> Drink plenty of water.

>> Reduce intake of fat, sugar, and refined flour.

>> Use healthier cooking methods such as baking, boiling, and steaming instead of frying.

>> Pay attention to your eating patterns that can lead to inactivity or overeating. This is where a nutritionist can help you modify your meals and the times you eat.

>> Participate in physical activities you enjoy, such as walking, bicycling, aerobics, or Zumba. Include strength training exercises to support muscle tone. Make sure your doctor gives you medical clearance to participate in any new type of exercise or rigorous exercise regimen.

Weight gain may be caused by your body's ability to store excess fluid in the tissues outside the blood vessels and lymphatic system. If you want to know if your weight gain is caused by fluid retention, look for the following symptoms:

- » Skin that feels firm or leaves small indentations after pressing on the swollen area

- » Swelling of the arms, wrist, legs, or ankle

- » Wristwatches, rings, bracelets, or even shoes fitting tighter than usual

- » Reduced flexibility in the wrist, fingers, hands, elbows, or legs

The following ideas can help you manage fluid retention:

- » Talk to your doctor and ask for a *diuretic* — medication that can get rid of the excess body fluid by increasing urination.

- » Reduce intake of sodium or salt in your diet. Remember that foods high in sodium don't always taste salty. Read the labels on any food that you purchase to determine the sodium content.

- » Weigh yourself daily at the same time and keep track of weight changes. Bring your weight log to your follow-up appointment with your doctor.

- » Participate in regular exercise during treatment to reduce weight gain.

- » Avoid standing for long periods because gravity will increase fluid to collect in your lower legs and feet.

- » Raise or elevate your feet above the level of the heart as often as possible.

- » Avoid crossing your legs because it restricts blood flow.

- » Avoid wearing tight clothing and close-fitting footwear.

- » Ask your doctor if you will benefit from wearing support or compression stockings.

Dealing with Diarrhea

Diarrhea can be a common symptom experience after cancer treatments. Sometimes the diarrhea may disappear after a few days, but it may go on for several weeks after your treatment. It's not only uncomfortable but can make you feel weak and tired and can lead to weight loss. Diarrhea can also cause you to become dehydrated. You must drink plenty of fluids to prevent dehydration.

WARNING

If your diarrhea is excessive (three or more loose stools within 24 hours), you must tell your doctor or nurse. You may also ask them about soothing creams to apply around your anus to prevent soreness or skin breakdown.

TIP

The following tips will help you to control diarrhea:

>> Eat smaller meals and more snacks.

>> Avoid fatty foods. These include fried foods and foods that are greasy or covered in gravy, which can make diarrhea worse.

>> Avoid milk, butter, ice cream, and cheese. Even if your diarrhea isn't caused by *lactose intolerance* (difficulty processing the sugar lactose, found in dairy products), stay away from these foods during a bout with diarrhea. Diarrhea can cause you to develop a temporary sensitivity to dairy foods.

>> Avoid foods that cause excess gas. Although it is important to eat large amounts of fruits and vegetables daily, when diarrhea strikes you should avoid foods that can increase intestinal gas, until you're feeling better. Those foods include beans, broccoli, cabbage, salads, spinach, and cauliflower.

>> Try low-fiber, starchy foods such as white bread and rice, pasta, and potatoes without their skins.

>> Avoid alcohol and caffeine drinks. Caffeine and alcohol act as *diuretics,* meaning they dehydrate you, or cause you to lose fluids.

>> Avoid sorbitol and other artificial sweeteners (Equal, Splenda, and similar products). Artificial sweeteners can have a laxative effect on your digestive system. So avoid sugarless candy and gum, diet soft drinks, and sugar substitutes.

>> Drink plenty of fluids to prevent dehydration.

>> Ask your doctor if anti-diarrheal drugs are appropriate.

>> Eat the following:

- Boiled potatoes

- Toast

- Plain crackers such as saltines

- Pretzels

- Baked chicken without any skin or fat

Chapter **17**

Cancer Treatment, Fertility, and Sexuality

"Will I be able to get pregnant, or will I be able to father a child?" These are often the thoughts in the minds of young women and men who are diagnosed with breast cancer before having children. Unfortunately, doctors may not always have the answers about what your fertility will be like after breast cancer treatment.

Fertility preservation is always an option. New innovations in fertility procedures allow the harvesting of eggs in a woman and the collection of sperm from a man to be completed within seven days. No longer does it take weeks or months to preserve your fertility prior to breast cancer treatment — don't let anyone tell you otherwise. You are of course focused on treating or getting a cure for your breast cancer, but you can have the best of both worlds by getting your treatment in timely fashion and having a baby after treatment. If that's what you want, you owe it to yourself to be happy and fulfilled.

This chapter provides you with information about who is at a baseline risk for infertility and which breast cancer treatments can increase infertility. Pay attention to the treatments available for infertility that include alternative therapies and traditional medicine discussed here. Embracing holistic approaches to health and wellness can increase your opportunity to regain your health, normal physical and sexual functions (including intercourse and pregnancy), and well-being.

Infertility and Breast Cancer

Infertility is the term used when a woman can't get pregnant or keeps having miscarriages. It affects one in eight couples of reproductive age in the United States and may be due to problems either in the man or woman.

Women are born with a specific number of eggs, and a woman's eggs begin to decline after the age of 32. At age 35 or older the rate of follicle loss accelerates, resulting in fewer and poorer quality eggs, making conception more difficult. A *follicle* is the sac that contains the egg, fluid, and supporting cells that are essential for pregnancy. During a woman's life the number of follicles gradually decreases, due to the process of degeneration or aging. The reduction of eggs in the ovaries eventually results in *menopause,* a naturally occurring biological process that happens 12 months after your last menstrual cycle and heralds the end of having menstrual periods altogether. Menopause typically occurs during a woman's 40s or 50s.

Infertility is a known side effect of cancer therapies. Breast cancer and cancer therapies can affect sexual health (including functioning and fertility) and sexual well-being (including feelings of desire, pleasure, sexuality, and so on). Breast cancer patients may face different fertility issues, including difficult fertilization after cancer, infertility, or impaired *fecundity* — your ability to produce offspring — along with compounded psychosocial distresses.

General causes of infertility

Table 17-1 outlines the major medical factors affecting fertility in cancer patients.

TABLE 17-1   **Medical Causes of Infertility in Cancer Patients**

Males	Females
Azoospermia, germ cell failure	Cancer or tumors
Cancer or tumors	Chromosome defects
Chromosome defects	Depletion of oocytes
Damage to pelvic nerves	Early menopause, amenorrhea
Hormone imbalance	Endometriosis
Infection or STD	Hormone imbalance
Lack of ejaculation	Infection or STD
Medications	Ovulatory disorder

Males	Females
Retrograde ejaculation	Medications
Sperm duct defects	Systemic diseases
Systemic diseases	Tubal disease
Testosterone deficiency	Uterine factor
Undescended testes	
Variocele	

Table 17-2 lists social and other determinants for infertility in cancer patients.

TABLE 17-2 ## Social Determinants of Infertility in Cancer Patients

Social determinants	Other determinants
Access to healthcare	Age
Country of origin	Alcohol abuse
Country or region	Celiac disease
Culture and norms	Illegal drug use
Education	Obesity
Ethnicity	Other health problems
Family background	Overexposure to heat
Immigration status	Problems with intercourse
Income	Tobacco smoking
Insurance	Toxic substances
Labor force participation	Vitamin deficiency
Neighborhood conditions	
Quality of care	
Religion	

Fertility and cancer treatment

Chemotherapy can stop your ovaries from working temporary or permanently. Whether your infertility is temporary or permanent, the likelihood of becoming infertile depends on the type of chemotherapy medications used, the dose given, and your age. Some chemotherapy and hormonal therapy may cause depletion in number of oocytes (eggs), hormonal imbalance, premature ovarian failure (POF), or very early menopause. Some chemotherapy drugs are more likely than others to cause infertility.

The chemotherapy medications *most* likely to cause injury to your eggs and infertility include the following:

>> Busulfan

>> Carboplatin

>> Carmustine (BCNU)

>> Chlorambucil

>> Cisplatin

>> Cyclophosphamide (Cytoxan)

>> Dacarbazine

>> Doxorubicin (Adriamycin)

>> Ifosfamide

>> Lomustine (CCNU)

>> Mechlorethamine

>> Melphalan

>> Procarbazine

>> Temozolomide

Chemotherapy medications that are *less* likely to cause injury to your eggs and infertility include the following:

>> 5-fluorouracil (5-FU)

>> Bleomycin

>> Cytarabine

>> Dactinomycin

>> Daunorubicin

>> Fludarabine

>> Gemcitabine

>> Idarubicin

>> Methotrexate

>> Vinblastine

>> Vincristine

Hormonal medications *most* likely to cause injury to your eggs and infertility include the following:

>> Evista (chemical name: raloxifene)

>> Fareston (chemical name: toremifene)

>> Tamoxifen

Permanent infertility

Permanent infertility occurs mostly with higher doses of medications and older age. You are more likely to have permanent infertility if you receive chemotherapy while you are close to the age where you would naturally have menopause. This occurs because some chemotherapy medications injure the eggs in the ovaries, so that none is left after treatment. If this happens, you can no longer get pregnant, and you may have symptoms of menopause.

WARNING

Some women may stop having a period during chemotherapy but are still producing eggs and could still get pregnant. Therefore, it's best to always use a reliable contraception method while having chemotherapy, even if your periods do stop, because you *can* get pregnant. More to the point, chemotherapy itself can harm the baby and cause birth defects.

Temporary infertility

You will know that your infertility is temporary when your periods become irregular or stop during treatment but return back to normal after your treatment is over. This happens in about a one-third of all women whose menstrual periods stop because of chemotherapy. Sometimes it may take 6–12 months for the menstrual period to return to normal after chemotherapy treatment has ended.

REMEMBER

In general, the younger you are when having chemotherapy treatment, and particularly if you're under 35, the more likely it is that your menstrual period will return. Women over 35 are more likely to lose their fertility by having early menopause.

Early menopause

If you're having early menopause, your menstrual period may either become irregular or later stop completely. In addition, you can experience the following symptoms:

>> Hot flashes

>> Dry skin

>> Vaginal dryness

>> Loss of energy

>> Less interest in sex

>> Mood swings or feeling low

REMEMBER

Not all breast cancer treatments affect fertility. Breast surgery and radiation alone to treat breast cancer will have no physical effect on fertility and won't increase the risk of it.

How to help preserve your fertility

First, talk to your doctor about how breast cancer treatment may affect your fertility and how you might preserve your fertility during treatment.

TIP

Discussions between you and your doctor about fertility preservation are most effective when they occur before treatment begins. Fertility preservation techniques are most effective prior to cancer treatment. Additionally, professional counseling can provide effective solutions to cope with the emotional aspects of dealing with changes in your fertility.

Some women may get pregnant naturally after their cancer treatment, whereas other women find they are unable to have children after treatment. Your breast cancer diagnosis will push you to think about fertility earlier than you had planned. Just the thought that your treatment can possibly affect your ability to get pregnant can be difficult to cope with — sometimes even as difficult as your cancer diagnosis.

Doctors are interested in new ways of preserving fertility for women with breast cancer. Current research is ongoing to find out how well methods of fertility preservation work and how safe they are.

Tissue banking and fertility preservation

Tissue banking and fertility preservation can be solutions for woman or couples who wish to pursue pregnancy in a later age. For some cancer patients and survivors, especially young survivors, ova (eggs), embryo, and ovarian tissues banking can be helpful to achieve fertilization when ovarian failure occurs.

IVF (freezing embryos)

Nowadays, in vitro fertilization (IVF) is the most effective way of preserving fertility. Here's how it works: You take hormones to stimulate your ovaries to produce more follicles from the existing eggs. A doctor then removes the eggs and fertilizes them with the male sperm. If you don't have a male partner at this stage, you will have the option to use a donor's sperm. The eggs and the sperm create an embryo which can be frozen and stored. After completing breast cancer treatment, one or more of these fertilized eggs or embryos can be placed into your womb to determine whether this can result in a pregnancy.

Techniques to successfully harvest and store reproductive cells have vastly improved over the past two decades. Doctors don't yet know what the effect of increasing the hormones to harvest eggs will have on women with hormone-positive breast cancer. Researchers have been looking into the following different ways of doing IVF:

» Natural cycle IVF using no hormones. This is at the investigation stage and so far it hasn't been as successful as regular IVF.

» Collecting eggs from the ovaries using smaller doses of hormones.

» Testing different hormone therapies to stimulate the ovaries, including tamoxifen and aromatase inhibitors, either on their own or in combination with a lower dose of IVF hormones.

Fertility preservation is still an emerging discipline, but advances in medical procedures and technology in the last several years are now providing new options for patients. However, offspring resulting from in vitro fertilization (IVF) may carry a greater risk for autoimmune diseases as they grow up.

Egg freezing

Doctors can also remove and freeze a women's eggs. This is a method often used when the woman doesn't have a male partner and doesn't want to use donor sperm. Hormones are used to stimulate the ovaries to produce the eggs, which are collected and frozen. Later, when you want to use the eggs, they are thawed and injected with sperm for fertilization. Research has shown that freezing and thawing eggs can damage them and has not been very successful. Talk to your doctor about the options available to you.

Ovarian tissue freezing

Ovarian tissue freezing involves a small operation to remove some ovarian tissue, which is then frozen. The tissue is placed back into your body after your cancer treatment has completed. This is an emerging treatment and is in early stages of development. There is little evidence so far about how well this procedure works, but there have been reports of women having babies after this procedure.

Alternative complementary and alternative medicine fertility treatments

Increasingly, complementary and alternative medicine (CAM) is being used to treat a variety of gynecologic and infertility-related disorders, including ovarian (and testicular) malfunction due to cancer treatments, polycystic ovarian syndrome (PCOS), endometriosis, and idiopathic infertility. Acupuncture is the most common form of CAM used for patients undergoing IVF, and acupuncture and herbal supplement are the most commonly used CAM therapies for male factor infertility.

Dietary changes and lifestyle habits are important parts of complementary medicine to increase fertility. The following are dietary suggestions to increase fertility:

» Increase intake of foods rich in omega-3 fatty acids found in coldwater or fatty fish and vegetable oils. Omega-3 fatty acids are also necessary for the relaxation and contraction of muscles, blood clotting, digestion, cell division, and more. DHA in omega-3 fatty acids is vital for fetal brain development. Research has shown that pregnant moms who ingest dietary supplements of DHA omega-3 fatty acids have babies with fewer behavior problems, better language skills, and higher IQs.

» Pregnant women may be discouraged from eating fish because of the contamination of mercury, but they can substitute omega-3 fatty acids with alpha-linolenic acid, found in walnuts. One ounce of walnuts has as much omega-3 fatty acids as 3.5 ounces of salmon. Other sources include flax seed, soybeans, canola oil, and other seeds and nuts.

» Increase intake of seeds, green vegetables, and legumes to increase follicular development.

>> Avoid alcohol and caffeine because they can cause hormone imbalance. They're also dehydrating, and the loss of water in the body may make cervical mucus too thick. Water plays a key role in transporting hormones and developing follicles. It also helps thin out cervical mucus, which may make it a little easier for your partner's sperm (those little swimmers) to get to their goal.

>> Avoid acidic foods like meat and processed foods, which may make your cervical mucus hostile to sperm.

>> Eat lots of baby carrots, sprouts, and wheat grass to maximize your body's baby-making juices because they're alkaline and natural body mechanisms are in place to maintain normal PH with the right intake of nutrition.

Good clinical care practice for infertility

Healthy People 2020 (www.healthypeople.gov) has suggested employing a "life course" perspective to health promotion and disease prevention on fertility issues to examine the quality of life. Cancer organizations and advocates recommend sexual health intervention and fertility preservation in cancer patients.

According to the American Society of Clinical Oncology (ASCO), cancer doctors should discuss fertility concerns prior to cancer treatment — as early in treatment planning as possible. Researchers have also suggested that best practice will be to have a multidisciplinary team (including oncologists, nurses in the specialties of oncology and infertility, psychooncologist, reproductive endocrinology, and infertility specialists, andrologists, and embryologists) come together initially to develop a treatment plan and fertility concerns for the cancer patient.

The BETTER model approach

Hughes and Cohen in a 2004 paper suggested clinicians use the BETTER model approach when communicating with patients about sexual health issues. "BETTER" is an acronym for six elements:

>> **B:** *Bring* up the topic. Start with clinical questions and then move to relationship and fertility concerns.

>> **E:** *Explain* that sexuality and fertility are important parts of quality of life for many.

>> **T:** *Tell* patients about resources to address their concerns.

>> **T:** *Timing* is important to discussing sexuality and fertility issues. They might seem inappropriate now, but questions may come later; encourage questions at any time. Some patients and families who have concerns about fertility may consider the options of fertility preservation (discussed earlier in this chapter).

>> **E:** *Educate* patients about side effects of their cancer treatments and changes in sexuality and fertility.

>> **R:** *Record* discussions, assessments, interventions, and outcomes.

Given the greater burden of cancer among ethnic and minority populations, research and programs addressing the continuum of cancer care, including sexual health assessments, fertility screenings, and sexual health, are urgently needed. Cultural and religious beliefs and practices may also pose barriers to communicating and addressing fertility issues.

The emotional side of fertility issues

An Institute of Medicine report entitled "Cancer Care for the Whole Patient" underscores the importance of comprehensive care including sexual health and infertility care in promoting well-being. The 2011 Livestrong Cancer Policy Platform Federal Priority Report suggested that young adult cancer survivors face additional issues, including fertility, education, and career challenges.

TIP

Oncology organizations and advocates recommend addressing the physical and emotional side of fertility concerns in cancer patients. Solutions and discussion to address infertility may be more challenging among cancer patients, survivors, and families. To help in coping with the emotional side of fertility challenges, it is recommended that young survivors talk about their concerns and feelings with partners, supportive family members, spiritual leaders, and their healthcare team. Partners and other family members may also benefit from psychosocial care, counseling, and spiritual and supportive care to address the distress associate with fertility challenges.

Pregnancy and cancer

Research suggests that pregnancy after cancer does not trigger recurrence, even after breast cancer; nor do cancer and its treatments result in increased risk for the offspring of cancer patients (Peate M et al., 2009; Thewes B et al., 2003). However, appropriate medical care is advised for pregnant cancer survivors. Many younger cancer survivors have normal pregnancies and welcome very healthy babies into their lives. There are other risk factors that may exist. People of high paternal age may be susceptible to environmental chemicals and infection in general. Also, advanced age pregnancy may result in complications such as miscarriage, chromosomal anomalies, pre-eclampsia, Caesarean delivery, gestational trophoblast diseases, placenta previa and placental abruption during pregnancy, and preterm birth.

Here are a couple of fertility information resources:

>> Fertile Hope (www.fertilehope.org) provides information on fertility and support services to cancer patients and survivors whose medical treatments present the risk of infertility.

>> Living Beyond Breast Cancer (www.lbbc.org) provides information on fertility and various other topics important to breast cancer survivors.

Sexuality and Breast Cancer

Having a diagnosis of breast cancer and undergoing treatment will almost certainly affect how you feel about sex and intimacy. There are times when you will not feel like having sex or being intimate when you're dealing with breast cancer and treatment. On the other hand, perhaps you find that sex helps you feel more normal during a time when you feel unsure about yourself. How breast cancer affects you sexually will be unique to you.

Changes in sexuality and intimacy are often associated with physical changes, especially after breast surgery, which can make you less comfortable with your body. Other breast cancer treatments, such as chemotherapy, can change your hormone levels and may affect your sexual desire and response.

REMEMBER

You may also experience relationship issues. These often come from your partner worrying about how to express love physically and emotionally to you after treatment (especially after surgery). Often the experience of breast cancer can be a growth period for couples, especially when both partners are involved in the treatment decisions and post-care.

Physical effects of cancer treatment on sexuality

Sexual desire and pleasure can change after cancer and its treatment. It is common to have a loss of sex drive from cancer and its treatments. If you're experiencing a decrease or loss of sex drive, and it's creating stress and distress for you and your significant other, there are options that may help, including medication.

TIP

Don't keep such problems to yourself. It's a good idea to talk with your doctors about the problem and have them make recommendations about what the best choices are for you.

The physical impact of breast cancer can be permanent, such as the loss of the breast due to the mastectomy. The appearance of the surgical and radiation scars may influence a person's appearance, body image, sexual functioning, and intimacy, as well as the partner's attitudes and behaviors regarding intimacy and the marital relationship. If the symptoms are from chemotherapy and radiation, then they will likely improve over time as your body heals after the treatments. Cancer and its treatment can cause hormonal imbalance, decreased lubrication, tightening of the vaginal area, and painful sex. In addition, other illnesses like hypertension, diabetes, depression, and even habits such as cigarette smoking can affect sexuality.

Pain

Some survivors experience pain during sex. Pain during sex can happen during and after chemotherapy, which affects a woman's hormones, causing changes in the vaginal tissue (such as tightening, drying, and inflammation). Yeast infections are also common during chemotherapy, which can cause itching and discomfort. Several survivors may have chronic pain in their chests and shoulders after radical mastectomy. This may be improved by supporting these areas with pillows during intercourse. Also, to prevent discomfort, avoid positions where weight rests on the chest or arm.

Hormone changes

Chemotherapy can result in decreased estrogen levels and premature menopause because it can damage the ovaries and stop them from producing estrogen and progesterone. As a result, hot flashes, vaginal dryness, mood swings, and fatigue from interrupted sleep can affect your interest and enjoyment in sex. Decreased lubrication can make sexual intercourse uncomfortable or painful. Using a vaginal lubricant that is natural and free from glycerin and paraben can help to relieve vaginal dryness, making sex more comfortable and pleasurable. Glycerine (a sugar alcohol) and parabens can increase the growth of bacteria in the vagina and bring on yeast infections and urinary tract infections (UTIs).

You may also want to consider asking your doctor about medications such as antidepressants, vitamins, and other supplements that can help relieve menopausal symptoms.

TIP

Organic coconut oil can be used for vaginal dryness. It provides the following benefits:

>> It's natural and safe.

>> As a lubricant, it moisturizes and soothes the vaginal area.

> **»** It's cheap, making it a cost-effective alternative.

> **»** It's an antibacterial and antifungal and can prevent yeast infections.

> **»** It reduces pain during sex because it moisturizes and allows the vaginal wall to stretch.

WARNING

For some women who can no longer have children as a result of cancer treatment, sexual activity may be a reminder of this loss. They may shy away from sexual activity because it is too painful to know that sex will not result in pregnancy.

Depression and anxiety

It is common for women to feel depressed or anxious after treatment. Depression and anxiety can get in the way of being able to enjoy sex the way you normally did. You can talk to a family member or seek the help of a professional if the depression and anxiety are too overwhelming.

TIP

In such instances, you can call the CRISIS hotline at 800-784-2433. Remember: Seeking help is not a sign of weakness — it's a sign of strength.

Loss of self-esteem

Sometimes women blame themselves for having cancer. Some survivors may feel that they can't trust their ability to find partners who will honor them and protect them. As a result, they may feel a loss of self-confidence and self-esteem. Others may feel undeserving of their partner's expressions of love and affection. They may feel damaged, incomplete, or even ashamed. Remember, you are not to blame for having cancer. Cancer is the second most common illness in the United States.

Changes in body image

The most common sexual side effect from breast cancer treatment is feeling less attractive. If a breast is removed, a woman may feel insecure about whether her partner will accept her and still find her sexually pleasing. She may have scarring, weight gain, or decreased energy, which makes a woman feel less attractive.

TIP

Even if you don't *look* very different, you may *feel* very different after cancer, no matter what anybody tells you. You may feel more vulnerable or fragile. These feelings can affect your sexuality. Try to do at least one self-nurturing activity a week. For example, plan a lunch date with a good friend, get your hair done, or buy a new lipstick. Pamper yourself and do things that make you feel sexy.

Fear of abandonment

A cancer diagnosis can leave a woman feeling anxious and uncertain. Surgeries resulting in changes in physical appearance can make a person feel that they are no longer attractive to their partner. After suffering the loss of your health, it's understandable that you may become afraid of other losses. This fear can impact your connection to your partner. You may feel less attractive than you did before and worry that your partner will leave for someone else. Avoid testing your partner. Be clear and honest about what you are feeling, especially about your fears. Don't think you can "read" your partner's mind and avoid getting into past conflicts or sorrows — be in the present. An open and honest conversation with your partner can bring you closer together and decrease feelings of frustration, guilt, and loss. The increased communication between you and your partner is necessary to maintain a satisfying sexual relationship, creating a greater sense of connection.

TIP

If you have some fears of abandonment, you can try talking with your partner or spouse about your feelings. If this is too difficult, you might ask the help of someone close to your partner or spouse to share your feelings. Additionally, you and your partner may want to explore aspects of your intimate lives that increase your comfort and connection with each other, such as alternate sexual positions that put less pressure on the abdomen (for example, woman on top or side-by-side).

Need for self-protection

After cancer, it's common for a woman to feel vulnerable, as though her life is threatened. You may find that the need to protect and take care of yourself is more important than acting on your sexual desires. Therefore, getting well becomes a priority, and sexual activity gets put on hold at least for a while.

TIP

Try to hug and cuddle with your partner more. These acts of affection can be very comforting and help the healing process. Focus more on creating intimacy. Make dates, take baths together, and hold hands. Most importantly, find time to talk about your feelings about your body and each other. In time, you will be physically and emotionally ready to renew your sexual relationship.

Sexuality and intimacy

Sexuality and intimacy are vital to our health and well-being. *Sexuality* involves more than you probably think. It can include sexual thoughts, fantasies, desires, attitudes, beliefs, values, practices, or activities alone or with a partner. For cancer survivors, a healthy sex life and sense of connection to another are especially important forms of expression that help relieve distress and promote healing.

Research shows that approximately one-half of women who have been treated for breast cancer experience sexual dysfunction (National Cancer Institute, 2006). Many survivors report that medical personnel seldom talk about sexual issues prior to or after treatment. Therefore, survivors often need information, support, and guidance in helping them feel normal about their sexual concerns, as well as to recover their sexuality.

TIP

You (and your partner) can talk with your doctor about your sexual concerns. If you feel uncomfortable talking with you doctor, you might first try talking with a nurse.

Cancer affects a woman's total being, including her body, mind, and spirit. A cancer diagnosis, surgery, and treatments can change your physical functioning along with your desire for sex and affect intimacy. This is particularly true with breast cancer survivors because the physical and emotional effects are further influenced by society's perceptions of beauty. In our culture, breasts are often viewed as a basic part of femininity and womanhood.

Sex after cancer

This section discusses the physical, emotional, and social impact of breast cancer on sexuality and offers recommendations for increasing your sexual satisfaction after cancer treatment. Sometimes women feel ashamed or guilty talking about sex, but sex is a normal and healthy part of life. It's natural to want to have an active and satisfying sex life.

TIP

Think back to how your partner has responded to you in the past about intimate issues such as your sex life together. Honest discussions about sex can be difficult even between partners who have been together for many years. If you don't feel comfortable talking to your partner about sex yet, these are a few things that you can do to enhance sexual intimacy:

>> Plan a date.

>> Have dinner at your favorite restaurant.

>> Go watch the sunset on the beach and let your partner know that you enjoy their company.

>> Talk about your first date.

>> Give your partner a massage or back rub.

>> Touch, cuddle, and kiss more.

>> Dress to help the mood. Sexy negligée and/or underwear can help a breast cancer survivor and her partner feel aroused. Sexy clothing can also help you feel more confident, especially if you're self-conscious about a scar or surgical site.

Talking to your partner about sex

It may be helpful to ask your partner questions about their feelings so that you're not assuming how they feel. Here are some questions you might consider asking:

>> How do you feel about my body after cancer?

>> What are some of the things that have felt good to you during sex?

>> Is there anything you would like to know about my experience with sex since having cancer?

>> Do you have any questions that you would like to have answered by a doctor or nurse?

Questions to ask myself

And here are some questions you should consider asking yourself:

>> How has cancer affected my feelings about my body?

>> How do I think my partner feels about my body now?

>> Have I ever asked my partner how they feel about my body?

>> What are some of the things that feel good to me during sex?

>> What are some things that don't feel good to me during sex?

>> What are some things I would like my partner to know about my experience with sex?

>> What kind of help would I like to get from my partner?

>> What questions do I want to ask my doctor or nurse about how my treatment has affected my experience with sex?

>> How do I feel about changes in my sexuality and sexual activities? What can I do to make the experience more pleasurable?

TIP

It's common for some survivors to lose interest in sex during the first six months to a year after diagnosis. If you continue to have the side effects of treatment and have lost interest in having sex or engaging in sexual activities, talk to your doctor and ask for suggestions on managing these side effects and improving sexual well-being.

Dating after cancer

Dating after cancer can be a challenge. Single women experience more or less the same challenge as women who are not single: depression, loss of self-esteem, changes in body image, fear of abandonment or rejection, and the need for self-protection. Women who are single may be nervous, fearful, or even hesitant about starting a new relationship. Their chief concern about dating might be, "Should I tell the person I am dating (or will date) that I had cancer, and if so, when?" A major concern of sharing this information is, "Will I be rejected once the person is aware that I am a cancer survivor?" The possibility of rejection is real, but it's important to not let the fear of rejection stop you from dating altogether. Fear could lead to withdrawal, isolation, increased anxiety, and depression.

Other difficult issues you may want to discuss with a new partner include your desire for children/parenting, whether or not you are able to bear children after the cancer, and the possibility of recurrence or the cancer coming back. Some new partners may also need to be reassured that cancer is not contagious.

Here are some ideas you can try:

>> Start working on other areas of your social life besides dating and sex. You might join a club or organization and connect with friends to increase your social gatherings and fun activities.

>> Make a list of your good points and focus on what you bring to a relationship.

>> Make a list of what you want your new partner to bring to the relationship.

>> Try not to let cancer be an excuse for not dating or trying to meet people.

>> You don't have to tell a new date about your cancer right away. This is your choice.

>> Practice what you will say to someone if you're worried about how they will handle it. Try to think about how they might react and be ready with a response.

>> Think about dating as a learning process with the goal of having a social life you enjoy. Not every date has to be a "success." If some people don't show interest in dating you (which can happen with or without cancer), that's okay because when the right relationship comes along, you will know it.

>> Remember that not all dates are for "keeps." Some dates can be for a few social and fun activities.

>> Wait until you feel a sense of trust and friendship before you're ready to have sex. Sex is fully under your control!

Chapter **18**

Making Healthy Lifestyle Changes

"An unhealthy habit is easy to develop and hard to live with; a healthy habit is harder to develop but easier to live with," says Dr. Rani Whitfield, a board-certified family physician with a certificate of added qualification (CAQ) in sports medicine. Many individuals use marijuana, drink alcohol, and smoke cigarettes to deal with anxiety, depression, stress at work, or family problems.

How do you know if you have anxiety or depression? The inability to relax, sleep, or even find joy out of life are sure ways to know. You must learn how to form healthy habits by replacing the bad ones. Healthy habits give you the benefit of good health, stamina, and a better quality of life.

Healthy Lifestyle Changes to Lose Weight

Anyone can learn healthy habits if they want to. It's not easy, but it certainly can be done — by anyone. There are several rules of thumb around the process of changing behaviors:

» **Change your mind.** You have the power to change your mind-set. Yes, you can do it. It typically takes 45–90 days to form a new habit. *Stick with it.* Remember that an unhealthy habit is attractive because it gives instant self-gratification, but you will pay for it later. When you form a healthy new habit, it means that you put off instant self-gratification to get the much bigger payoff in the future. Believe in yourself and your ability to change, and you will.

» **Be realistic.** Look at how your emotions and behaviors affect your health. What are your self-destructive behaviors? Work on avoiding negative self-talk. Always look at the cup as half full instead of half empty. Journaling, visualization, and positive affirmations can help improve your self-esteem and make your goals more attainable. Speaking of . . .

» **Set attainable goals.** Divide every large goal into smaller goals to make it realistic and attainable.

Define your ultimate goal. Then break it into smaller goals and write them all down with an action plan to hold yourself accountable. Setting attainable goals will help you to review the progress you're making toward the ultimate goal — and will keep you motivated.

Think of your new habit as a *replacement* instead of *deprivation*. Instead of eating a slice of cake or potato chips, eat a piece of fruit, such as an apple, banana, or grapes. If you want to lose weight, focus on your summer vacation on the beach wearing a bikini.

» **Reward yourself.** Treat yourself to a day in the spa, massage, new outfit, pair of shoes, and so forth. Keep believing in yourself with self-affirmation daily.

» **Set up a support system.** Even though you are responsible for your own success, having support from your friends and family can increase your commitment to achieving your goal. Tell someone you trust about your goal and how you're planning to accomplish it. For example, you can give them an update on the foods that you're no longer eating. You can tell them about your new meal plan, exercise regimen, and so on. This can help keep you accountable, because you won't want to disappoint them. Let your family and friends know how important it is for you to have their support.

» **Make healthier choices.** Empty the pantry and refrigerator of any junk foods immediately. Restock with fresh fruits, vegetables, lean proteins, and whole grains. It's important that you plan out a few go-to healthy meals too, so you can stock up. Always have things like snack-size baby carrots, nuts, and yogurt that you can easily take when you are on the run.

>> **Keep moving.** The best way to burn calories is through exercise.

TIP

You burn the most calories when you exercise in the morning before breakfast. When you wake up in the morning after fasting all night, your body doesn't have a choice but to burn stored fat for energy, thus your weight loss will be higher.

>> **Allow a "cheat" once in a while.** If you're regularly exercising and avoiding concentrated sweets, and then you go to a birthday party, go ahead and have a slice of cake. Because of your commitment to exercising and eating healthy, it's okay to have a slice or eat a crazy meal once a week.

>> **Replace watching television and electronic games with exercise.**

Chapter 17 talks more about weight loss strategies.

Healthy Lifestyle Changes for Anxiety and Depression

Lifestyle changes are powerful tools to overcome depression and relieve anxiety. If you have moderate or severe anxiety and/or depression, we advise you to seek medical care along with implementing lifestyle changes.

This section discusses broad lifestyle changes that can help anxiety and depression.

Exercise

Exercise is vital for maintaining mental fitness and reducing stress. Research has shown that exercise is very effective at reducing fatigue and improving concentration, alertness, and overall cognitive function. This confers a benefit, especially when you feel like stress has depleted your energy or ability to mentally focus.

Exercise stimulates the body to produce serotonin and endorphins, which are chemicals in the brain (neurotransmitters) that alleviate depression. Many researchers have found that exercise is effective in elevating mood and reducing symptoms of depression. Anxiety symptoms are improved with relaxation exercises such as yoga, tai chi, and mindful movement. Improved self-esteem is a key psychological benefit of regular physical activity.

When you exercise, the endorphins your body releases interact with receptors in your brain to reduce your perception of pain and trigger a positive feeling in the body, similar to that of morphine. That "euphoric" feeling that follows an intense physical workout, or *runner's high,* can have you energized and enjoying a positive outlook on life. Endorphins produced in the brain, spinal cord, and many other parts of your body are released in response to neurotransmitters.

Participating in an exercise program can help in the following ways:

>> Reducing stress

>> Increasing self-esteem

>> Warding off anxiety and depression

>> Boosting self-confidence

>> Improving sleep

>> Creating a sense of independence and empowerment

>> Enhancing social connection

>> Improving communication and relationships

Additional exercise benefits include the following:

>> Strengthening the heart

>> Lowering blood pressure

>> Improving muscle tone and strength

>> Strengthening and building bones

>> Reducing body fat

>> Increasing libido and sex drive

>> Making you look fit and healthy

Easy exercises for anxiety and depression

Any form of exercises can help depression. However, you may find that moderate exercises are more sustainable. Here are some moderate exercises that provide benefits without being too strenuous:

>> Walking

>> Dancing

>> Biking

- » Jogging
- » Playing tennis
- » Yoga
- » Zumba
- » Low-impact aerobics
- » Swimming
- » Gardening
- » Golf (walking instead of using the cart)
- » Doing housework, especially sweeping, mopping, or vacuuming

Moderate exercises for anxiety and depression

The following types of exercise involve a little more effort but are especially good for relieving anxiety:

- » **Light jogging:** This is one of the best ways to improve your anxiety. Many people don't like jogging, but if you try it, you'll find that the more you jog, the easier it gets and the less anxiety you will have.

- » **Swimming:** This is more intense than walking, but you can still go at your own pace. The resistance of the water will strengthen and tone your muscles, giving you a good workout.

- » **Yoga:** Besides being physically demanding, yoga also teaches better breathing habits, which helps in reducing active anxiety.

More intense exercises for anxiety and depression

The following activities are a little more intense, but worth it. They can help fight anxiety and depression even more:

- » **Achieving daily healthy living:** This is when you find ways daily to increase your physical activity and utilize exercise as a therapeutic way to help you cope daily with depression and anxiety. Examples might include biking to work, hiking over the weekend, walking to the bus stop, or anything you can do to live a more active lifestyle.

- » **Joining a gym — and actually going regularly:** You can participate in mild, moderate, or intense exercises. All of these types can help manage anxiety and depression. There is no limit to the number of exercises you can do in a gym, and you can advance in intensity at your own pace.

>> **Long-distance jogging:** When you get to the final destination, this is where you experience the "runner's high" — that massive rush of endorphins that is great at controlling anxiety and depression.

Quitting Bad Habits Like Smoking, Drinking, and Drug Abuse

A *habit* is a behavior that is practiced over and over again — just as it can be *unpracticed* over and over again. Why smoke? Why drink alcohol? Why use illicit drugs? Many individuals provide the following reasons for indulging in these behaviors:

>> Curiosity or peer pressure, especially in the teen years

>> Family influences, if individuals in the household are smoking, drinking, or using illicit drugs

>> Already using other illicit drugs or participating in other bad habits

>> Stress relief

>> Boredom or just for something to do

Quitting bad habits first starts from you acknowledging that you have a problem or have been practicing unhealthy behaviors and want to make a change. Making the decision for your health and being motivated to make that change are the keys to being successful at quitting bad habits. This section discusses how to stop those bad habits and be a healthier you.

Quitting smoking

Quitting smoking starts with developing a determination to quit. Understanding the short-term and long-term benefits of quitting smoking in terms of your emotional, physical, spiritual, and social needs is critical for your determination to quit. Write down why you want to quit smoking. Keep what you wrote handy when you are tempted start back smoking or when you have the cravings for a cigarette.

Benefits of quitting smoking include the following:

>> Decreased risk of cancer, lung disease, heart attacks, stroke, and vision problems

>> Longer life expectancy

- ›› Lower risk of miscarriage or of having a baby born with a low birth weight
- ›› Better smelling breath and whiter teeth
- ›› Better smelling body and clothes
- ›› Saving money
- ›› No more yellowing of the fingernails and fingers
- ›› Heightened sense of smell and taste
- ›› Better skin color and texture
- ›› Easier breathing
- ›› Better healing when you have surgery
- ›› No longer exposing others to secondhand smoke
- ›› Greater acceptance from potential employers, or landlords, or car buyers

Quitting smoking requires both physical and emotional treatments. Some treatments are designed to treat the withdrawal symptoms that are associated with quitting smoking. Here are some of the main treatments:

- ›› Nicotine replacement therapy (NRT) may be given in patch, chewing gum, lozenge, or spray form.
- ›› Bupropion (Zyban or Wellbutrin) is a medication traditionally used for depression that can help with nicotine cravings.
- ›› Varenicline (Chantix) is a medication that decreases withdrawal symptoms as well as nicotine's effect on the brain.
- ›› Nortriptyline is an antidepressant that may help increase the chance of success when quitting smoking.
- ›› Clonidine is a medication traditionally used to decrease high blood pressure that may help with quitting smoking.

Psychological support is also important. This kind of support can include the following:

- ›› Talk therapy
- ›› Telephone-based counseling
- ›› Support groups
- ›› Classes or programs for quitting smoking

HIP-HOP DOC'S (DR. RANI WHITFIELD) BEST HABITS FOR HEART HEALTH

- Engaging in consistent exercise, 30 minutes a day, 7 days a week

- Quitting smoking

- Taking meds faithfully if you currently need them for high blood pressure, diabetes, high cholesterol, or heart disease

TIP

There are mobile apps (such as Quitter and Butt Out) that track your daily progress (such as how much money you've saved, or how many hours of life gained). These can provide positive reinforcement when you're feeling temptation.

Limiting or avoiding alcohol

There's nothing wrong with enjoying a social drink or a glass of wine at an occasional meal. Doing so may even confer health benefits that can prolong your life. Research shows that drinking moderate amounts of alcohol may protect healthy adults from developing coronary heart disease.

But when people use alcohol as a stress reliever to escape personal, social, emotional and physical pressures, alcoholism or abuse can result. When more alcohol is consumed than your body can handle, you can begin suffering from many illnesses.

Alcohol affects the body in the following ways:

>> **Brain:** It interferes with how brain cells communicate, causes disruption in mood and behavior, and increases difficulty in coordination and concentration.

>> **Heart:** It can damage the heart and cause the following:

- Arrhythmias, or irregular heartbeat

- Stroke

- High blood pressure

- Cardiomyopathy (stretching and drooping of heart muscle)

>> **Liver:** The liver is the organ that has to process and break down the alcohol you drink. Heavy drinking of alcohol can cause injury to your liver, including the following:

- Cirrhosis is the end stage of liver failure when the liver tissue is replaced with fibrosis.

- Steatosis, or fatty liver.

- Alcoholic hepatitis is inflammation of the liver (hepatitis) due to excessive intake of alcohol.

- Fibrosis is thickening and scarring of connective tissue that is often caused by injury.

» **Pancreas:** Alcohol causes the pancreas to become inflamed, called *pancreatitis.* The inflammation in the pancreas leads to erroneous release of digestive enzymes that cause it to begin to digest itself. Pancreatitis can be life-threatening and causes severe pain in the stomach area.

» **Cancer:** Alcohol can increase your risk of developing certain cancers of the

- Mouth

- Esophagus

- Throat

- Breast

- Liver

- Bladder

» **Immune system:** Alcohol weakens your immune system, making it easier for you to develop disease or infection. Heavy drinkers are more at risk for contracting respiratory viruses, pneumonia, and tuberculosis than people who don't drink too much.

Treatment for alcoholism

Treatment can only begin when the alcoholic accepts that there is a problem and help is needed to stop drinking. Alcoholism is a disease and is quite curable, but you must be motivated to change. There are three stages of treatment:

» **Detoxification (detox):** This stage may require support from a medical facility because detox can result in withdrawal seizures, hallucinations, delirium tremens (DT), and in rare cases even death.

» **Rehabilitation:** This stage involves counseling and medication to give the recovering alcoholic the skills needed for coping and maintaining sobriety. This stage is often done in-patient or out-patient.

» **Maintenance:** This stage involves the regular attendance of Alcoholics Anonymous (AA) meetings and getting a sponsor.

Overcoming drug abuse

If you have a desire to obtain or increase your use of substances in order to function, then the reality is you have a problem with drug abuse. Drug abuse affects your body and mind and creates physical drug dependence.

Dependence on the drug is not required for drug use to be considered drug abuse.

The effects of drug abuse are both physical and psychological.

The most common physical effects of drug abuse include the following:

>> Sleep changes

>> Decreased memory

>> Decreased cognition

Other common physical effects from drug abuse include the following:

>> Abnormal vital signs like respiration, heart rate, and blood pressure

>> Heart failure

>> Liver disease

>> Nausea, vomiting, diarrhea, and stomach pain

>> Chest or lung pain

>> Skin cool and sweating or hot and dry

>> Diseases such as hepatitis B or C, or HIV from needle-sharing

>> Impotence

>> More frequent illnesses

>> Frequent hangovers and blackouts

Here are the two main psychological effects of drug abuse:

>> Drug craving can cause you to be preoccupied with getting the drug, especially getting the money and finding where the drug can be purchased.

>> It increases mood changes and causes increased anxiety or depression due to side effects of the drug.

FOOD-HANDLING SAFETY TIPS FOR BREAST CANCER SURVIVORS

If you are a breast cancer survivor and actively receiving treatment, you may be at risk for foodborne illness because your immune system is not as strong to fight off a disease.

The following are safe-food handling tips to follow:

- **Clean:** Wash hands and surfaces often.
- **Separate:** Separate raw meat and poultry from ready-to-eat foods.
- **Cook:** Cook food to the right temperatures.
- **Chill:** Chill raw meat and poultry as well as cooked leftovers promptly (within two hours).
- **Store:** Make sure you're storing food and beverages properly and using them within recommended storage guidelines.

Cooking food at the right temperature is very important. Heat kills bacteria at the right temperature. You must also allow a rest time after the food is removed from the heat source such as a stove or grill. You can check out a handy chart of safe cooking temperatures for many kinds of food at www.foodsafety.gov/keep/charts/mintemp.html.

Other psychological drug abuse side effects include these:

- ›› Aggressiveness or irritability
- ›› Selfishness
- ›› Hopelessness
- ›› Lack of pleasure from previously enjoyed activities
- ›› Pressuring others into doing drugs

Maintaining Good Nutrition and Diet

Nutrition is the intake of food, considered in relation to the body's dietary needs and regular physical activity. Good nutrition is the intake of an adequate, well-balanced diet according to the dietary needs of the body. Poor nutrition can lead to reduced immunity, increased susceptibility to disease, impaired physical and mental development, and reduced productivity.

Many people take one or more dietary or nutritional supplements either every day or occasionally. Today's dietary supplements include vitamins, minerals, herbals and botanicals, amino acids, enzymes, and many other products. Dietary supplements may come in the form of tablets, capsules, powders, energy bars, and drinks. The most common dietary supplements are vitamins C, D, and E; minerals like calcium and iron; herbs such as Echinacea and garlic; and specialty products like glucosamine, probiotics, and fish oils.

When you select a dietary supplement, you'll notice the Supplement Facts panel on the packaging that lists the contents, amount of active ingredients per serving, and other added ingredients (like fillers, binders, and flavorings). Serving size is often suggested by the manufacturer, but your doctor may recommend a different amount that is appropriate for you.

REMEMBER

Dietary supplements should *not* take the place of the variety of foods that are necessary for a healthy diet. Supplements are meant to be just that — supplements. Dietary supplements can be an addition to a healthy diet that will help you get essential nutrients, but mustn't be used as a substitute or replacement.

Foods that can increase or lower estrogen

Most women in menopause dread the dry skin, thinning hair, and vaginal dryness that comes when your body has less estrogen. Wanting to replace your estrogen is a normal reaction to a substance that is lacking in your body. But in the case of having a history of breast cancer, you have to be very careful and reduce the amount of estrogen that you can get in foods and skin care products. Many breast cancer survivors ask us, "What can I eat?" and the response is often: a healthy, balanced meal with lots of fruits and vegetables.

However, if you breast cancer was estrogen-receptor-positive, you will want to ensure that you avoid foods that are high in estrogen and that you eat a lot of foods that lower or block estrogen. Several research studies have shown that when you eat a plant-based diet that is rich in phytoestrogens, your estrogen levels in your body will increase. Cruciferous vegetables have high levels of phytochemicals that block the production of estrogen in your body and they are great to cook and even eat raw. Table 18-1 shows some common foods that can increase or decrease estrogen in your body.

TABLE 18-1   **Foods That Affect Estrogen Levels**

Foods That Increase Estrogen (phytoestrogens)	Foods That Decrease Estrogen (cruciferous vegetables)
Seeds: flaxseeds and sesame seeds	Arugula
Fruit: prunes, apricots, oranges, strawberries, peaches, many dried fruits	Broccoli
Vegetables: yams, carrots, alfalfa sprouts, kale, celery	Cabbage
Soy products: soy protein powder, soy milk, tofu, miso soup, soy yogurt, soy veggie burger	Brussels sprouts
Dark rye bread	Bok choy
Legumes: lentils, peas, pinto beans	Kale
Olives and olive oil	Collard greens
Chickpeas	Turnips
Culinary herbs: turmeric, thyme, sage	Rutabagas
Multigrain bread	Cauliflower
Black bean sauce	Horseradish
Pistachio	Wasabi
Black licorice	Watercress

TIP

Animal products such as poultry and meats can increase the estrogen levels in your body if the farmers use hormones to raise the animals. Read labels and eat meats and poultry that are free from hormones.

Cooking and food preparation

How you prepare your foods is a probably central part of your lifestyle. We learn to cook from our families and our culture. There are some cooking styles that reduce the nutrients and vitamins in food, such as cooking vegetables for a long time.

TIP

You may find that vegetables taste great and keep their freshness, color, vitamins, and minerals if cooked for less than ten minutes. Be creative with mixing spices and vegetables. Add your favorite spices or try using lemon, salsa, curry, thyme, oregano, cumin, and ginger.

Portion control is key. Too much of anything isn't good. Table 18-2 lists some handy ways of thinking about portions of different kinds of foods.

TABLE 18-2   **Recognizing Proper Portions of Various Foods**

Food	How to Think of a Portion
3 oz. meat	Deck of playing cards
Apple	Tennis ball
1 oz. cheese	One egg
1/2 cup ice cream	Tennis ball
Cup of mashed potatoes, cooked pasta, rice, veggies	A fist
1 oz. nuts or candy	Filling a palm
Pancake	Compact disc
Serving of fish	Small checkbook
2 tablespoons butter, margarine, cream cheese, peanut butter	Two thumbs (a woman's thumb is approximately the size of 1 tablespoon, from the tip of the thumb to the first knuckle)
Cookie	Half a yo-yo
Muffin	Tennis ball

Weight Control and Activity

Here are some helpful ways of staying active and controlling your weight:

» Use the stairs rather than the elevator.

» Take a 10-minute break at work to stretch or take a quick walk.

» Walk with workmates at lunch.

» Go dancing with your spouse or friends.

» Walk an extra lap around the mall.

» Park your car a little farther and walk the extra distance.

» Lift some light weights or do a few sit-ups or jumping jacks during TV commercial breaks.

Weight control is key to the prevention and or maintenance of many cancers as well as other chronic medical diagnoses such as diabetes, heart disease, stroke, and hypertension. Weight control becomes more challenging as we age and our metabolism slows. We're also exposed to food advertisements that make larger portions seem tastier and the better choice. In the last century, as technology has advanced, we have become increasingly inactive, and our bodies and minds have suffered for it.

The good news is that the body has an incredible capacity to adjust and bounce back — emotionally, mentally, and physically. Lifestyle changes are never easy, but it's possible to transition toward healthier ways without relapsing back into old behavior.

Concrete steps to take toward healthier lifestyle changes

Try the following to improve your lifestyle and make it healthier:

>> **Be more aware of calorie intake:** Look at labels and make a log of what foods you eat, at least in the beginning. You might be surprised at how quickly you become an expert at this.

>> **Balance calorie intake with physical activity:** Make sure you set realistic goals for yourself and do activities you prefer, such as walking, biking, dancing, cleaning, or gardening.

>> **Plan your exercise routine to gradually increase over a period of several weeks.** Increase what you do and the length of time you exercise. Don't be afraid to try different activities. Whatever exercise activities you decide to do need to be done for at least 30–45 minutes four or five times a week to lose weight. To maintain ideal weight, exercise activities can be done about three times a week.

REMEMBER

>> **If you have a previously diagnosed medical condition, discuss your activity plan with your doctor before you start.** It's a good idea to talk with your doctor when starting any new diet or exercise routine in order to have a starting point for your medical status and realistic goals for your new lifestyle changes. Information is power. There's no need to fear it.

>> **Exercise at lunch by yourself or with coworkers.** Doing so is an opportunity to interact, reflect, stay fit, and manage stress. At least 15 minutes of uninterrupted activity is needed to get and keep your heart rate up for the best physical effect.

>> **Increase fruit and vegetable intake over a period of weeks to help adjust to healthier eating.** You may prefer trying different types of fruit and vegetables until you find the ones you like. Most restaurants have healthy choices — ask to see those items first. Some fruits and vegetables mix well together in salads and cooked side dishes, so experiment and find what works for you.

>> **Limit alcohol consumption.** Most alcoholic drinks have high sugar content, which becomes useless calories and carbohydrates in your body. Women should not have more than one alcoholic drink a day — any more than that puts women at risk for cancer or recurrence of cancer.

>> **Understand that low fat doesn't always mean low calorie.** For weight loss to be achieved, it's necessary to reduce calorie intake until a desired weight is achieved.

>> **Be aware of how much juice or soda you're consuming.** Most sodas and juices are full of calories and carbohydrates that become sugar in the body. However, there are many diet and reduced sugar options. Alternate diet soda with your use of regular soda drinks while trying to decrease soda intake. And be careful of flavored exercise water. Some flavored waters have more sodium, and if they're being used in place of water, they can add more than 100 mg of sodium a day to your diet.

>> **Eat breakfast and have six small meals a day.** This will go a long way toward keeping healthy sugar levels in your body, which will reduce cravings and overeating.

>> **Eat out less and prepare more of your own foods.** This is the only way to actually have control over food intake and diet and how your food is prepared. Prepare for cravings by having snacks and alternate foods available in your pantry at home and on your desk at work. Carry a bottle of water and meals with you whenever you can in your car, lunch bag, or portable cooler.

>> **Stay hydrated.** Drinking water and liquids helps you cleanse from the inside. Filter your tap water and consider adding fruit or flavors like strawberry, citrus, cucumber, or even herbs and spices like fresh ginger and basil.

Quick meals to make for healthy living

Here are some easy ways to prepare good foods for on-the-go:

>> Make an English muffin pizza with pizza or spaghetti sauce and a reduced fat cheese such as mozzarella. Top with mushrooms, chopped onions, chopped green peppers, tomato slices, broccoli florets, avocado, lean meats (chicken and turkey), and so forth. Use your imagination. Whatever you like!

>> Top parmesan-flavored couscous (a type of pasta available in most grocery stores) with cooked chopped chicken and vegetables.

>> Top cooked linguini with marinara sauce and minced clams, lean meats, or vegetables.

>> Top mixed salad greens (wash carefully) with vegetables and cubed cheese of your choice. The lower in fat the cheese, the better for your health. Top with any low-fat dressing of your choice and be careful to look at the calories and carbohydrates. A cup of salad is a regular serving size. Remember that a serving of dressing is usually a tablespoon. Vinegar and vinaigrettes are

usually lower in calories, but it does depend on the items used. Try using lemon juice to give the salad more flavor.

REMEMBER

>> Cook a quick and easy chili using extra-lean ground beef or ground turkey breast, canned or cooked kidney beans, tomato sauce, chopped onion, canned chopped tomatoes, and chili seasoning.

Canned items often have loads of sodium and sugar, so it's important to read the labels and try to use fresh or frozen vegetables instead. It's usually best to cook the beans and tomatoes yourself.

>> Top mini bagels with peanut butter or cheese and a sliced apple.

>> Stuff whole wheat tortillas with black beans, lettuce, salsa, low-fat cheese, low-fat sour cream, and jalapeños (if you dare).

>> Microwave a potato and top it with broccoli, cauliflower, and cheese as a meal.

If you're not into meat, you can use substitutes that still have protein, such as soy or gluten products. Wheat gluten or gluten powder is usually canned or packaged and found in the Asian food item aisles of larger supermarkets. It's also found in Asian markets located in most communities.

Tofu, a soy product, can be found in most supermarkets now. It comes in a packed block form, is generally white in color, and comes in soft, firm, or hard textures. Tofu needs to be refrigerated.

Gluten and soy take on the flavor of the seasonings and oils they're cooked with. For truly flavorful meals using these items, the longer the tofu or gluten is marinated in the seasonings, the more flavor it will absorb.

WARNING

There is some controversy with using soy products. Soy does have estrogen in it, so cancer survivors need to speak with their physician about whether they should use soy products.

General Health Guidelines for Optimal Health

To end this chapter, here are some general guidelines for achieving and maintaining optimal health:

>> Wear sunscreen and protect yourself against skin cancer if you're going to be outdoors for more than 10 minutes. Also try wearing a hat and sunglasses to protect your face and eyes from the damaging effects of the sun.

» Talk to your doctor about screenings for skin cancer if you have unusual moles, notice changes in the size of moles, or develop itchy patches on your skin.

» Talk to your doctor about checking your hearing.

» If you experience allergies or shortness of breath, talk to your doctor about asthma.

» Keep up with regular visits to the dentist twice a year.

» Visit the optometrist every year.

» Get a physical exam every year and keep copies of your results so you have an accurate record of your physical health.

» If you're sexually active or 18 years of age and older, you should have regular Pap tests according to the guidelines in your country.

» If you're sexually active, you need to have a screening for sexually transmitted infections.

» If you're age 50 and older or have a history of colon cancer in your family, talk to your doctor about screenings for colon cancer.

» If you're overweight, talk to your doctor about screenings for diabetes.

TIP

Research shows that being overweight and avoiding physical activity can increase your chances of a cancer recurrence. The best ways to maintain a strong body and reduce weight gain are to eat a healthy diet and move your body. Body movements are fun ways to relieve stress. Walking, dancing (even at home), and gardening (with protective gloves) release endorphins, the chemicals in your body that act as natural painkillers and provide a feeling of happiness and well-being. Moving your body for at least 20 minutes, three times per week, can increase your energy and help you feel better.

5
The Part of Tens

Check out ten inspiring breast cancer survivors — real-life people telling their real-life stories.

Find ideas on how your friends and family can help you through this — and what not to do.

Discover inspiring and surprising ways in which life after cancer can be better than ever.

Chapter **19**

Ten Inspiring Breast Cancer Survivors

W e're going to get into some inspiration stories from breast cancer survivors in this chapter — some of them in their own personal words. But first, let's talk a little bit about survivorship itself.

Let's say you've completed surgery or chemotherapy and/or radiation. The surgeon told you that you heal well and have no wound complications. Or maybe you've completed the "red devil" combination of chemotherapy with four cycles of Adriamycin and Cytoxan followed by 12 weeks of Taxol. Or you completed five weeks of radiation, and the last week of the radiation, you received boost doses of radiation — and all of a sudden your breast got red, skin became discolored, or the skin is sloughing off to make way for new skin. Maybe you're currently taking endocrine therapy with tamoxifen or anastrozole, and the hot flashes are getting to you — or you're moody, or it hurts when you are having sex, or you just have no libido. Know that this too shall pass — there is a light at the end of the tunnel.

When we talk about survivorship, we break it into three categories:

>> **Acute survivorship:** This is just after getting the diagnosis of breast cancer. Women often experience "the shock" and immediately start thinking about life decisions.

>> **Transitional survivorship:** This comes just after initial treatment for breast cancer (whether surgery, chemotherapy, or radiation). You may be taking endocrine therapy for 5–10 years after treatment to reduce your recurrence risk. This is also the time when most women feel uneasy because their medical visits are not as frequent and they are taking less medication. Sometimes women may even equate not getting active treatment to increasing the chance of breast cancer coming back. You may also see a reduction in social support while you are struggling to get control over your symptoms or lifestyle. This transition into a "new normal" is not one that happens instantly; it's a process that comes with time, self-perseverance, objectivity, and self-discovery. The best therapy for this stage of survivorship is to engage in exercise (Zumba, sporting activities, and so forth), eat healthy, and focus on the renewed you.

>> **Extended survivorship:** You will continue to have follow-up visits for 5–10 years with your cancer doctor depending on whether you're on endocrine therapy. If you're not on endocrine therapy, you will continue your regular follow-up with your primary care or general practitioner. During this period you may have unresolved issues that are important to you, such as managing lingering side effects of breast cancer treatment and any perceived psychosocial stress.

REMEMBER

In addition, some patients worry that the primary care provider is inadequate to oversee the surveillance of breast cancer. Have no fear. The survivorship care plan that your cancer doctor provides to you at your transition back to your primary care provider will list the breast cancer surveillance recommendations and necessary screening activities that you should participate in.

Helen Hosein-Mulloon

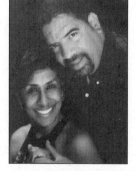

FIGURE 19-1:
Breast cancer survivor Helen Hosein-Mulloon.

Photo used with permission.

Helen Hosein-Mulloon (Figure 19-1) is a certified health coach, certified records analyst (CRA), and an information technology (IT) professional. She has worked in Trinidad and Tobago's energy sector for the past 28 years and has worked with leading multinational companies in different roles involving IT, facilities management, and records management. She is the current president of the Trinidad and Tobago Association of Records Managers and Administrators (ARMA) chapter.

Helen has volunteered with local cancer and multiple sclerosis societies for several years. She is a poet and a writer, plays piano, and is a globe-trotter, avid health enthusiast, devoted wife, and doting mother of 21-year-old aspiring arts journalist Kadeem and 16-year old artist and chef Marina. She has a grand-dog Cocker Spaniel named Snow.

Here is her story in her own words:

> Three days after my 40th birthday, I began chemotherapy. What seemed to be a routine checkup three months before turned into a diagnosis of triple negative stage II cancer in my right breast. My children were 14 and 9, and my husband worked a two-week rotation offshore. My own mother (a nonsmoker) was dead at 61 from lung cancer. Already diagnosed with multiple sclerosis two years earlier, I did not need another challenge.
>
> But my journey was laid out, a path I had to walk to a destination that I now see has made all the difference in my life.
>
> After 20 weeks of chemo, one month of daily radiation, a few falls, countless tear-filled nights, and lots of home-cooked meals from family, accompanied by hugs and love from friends and loved ones, I celebrated the end of treatment with a gluten-free Tinkerbell cake. My life, which seemed to be ending with that horrible diagnosis in August 2009, got a jolt in May 2010.
>
> As a family, we vacationed every year, and I decided to make lifetime memories over the next few years before the children went on to university. My focus was more on my life's purpose than the other things I had previously pursued.
>
> My children had to deal with a mother who is still battling critical illness issues. They had to grow up a little faster than their peers, but they are empathetic, warm young people as a result. My husband has been my rock, and without him, his support, and our shared faith, I would not be here.
>
> My favorite Biblical passage, Psalms 23, is still my comfort. I don't fear death — I've been at its doorstep and back. I fear not making my life count. God brought me to

a place where I still stand today: a better wife, a more devoted mother, an advocate for self-care, a volunteer to NGOs whose causes have impacted my life, a certified health coach, and a woman with a passion to help people be better and live healthier.

My mantra is to be a positive force to every person with whom I connect.

Linda Doyle

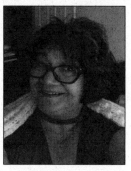

Linda Doyle (Figure 19-2) is a wife, mother, and grandmother. She works as a senior data management specialist.

My world changed at the beginning of 2013 when I was diagnosed with stage I invasive lobular cancer on my right breast through a routine mammogram. Thank God for the persistence of the radiologist who called me back for additional screening.

The first surgeon I went to see performed the biopsy but said I probably didn't have cancer so I was not too concerned at this point. When the results came back, he came into the examining room and blurted out, "Just as I suspected, you have breast cancer." I did not expect to hear that, especially since he had told me it was probably nothing. I was in shock. I looked over at my husband, and the look on his face was an expression I never want to ever see again.

It was important to me to get all my questions answered and have trust in my doctor. I wasn't feeling it. I decided to call Johns Hopkins Bayview Breast Center for a second opinion. I immediately knew this is where I was meant to be after meeting my surgeon. When I walked into the examining room, the nurse saw my fear, looked straight into my eyes, and said, "This is not a death sentence."

The doctor answered all my questions, told me what needed to be done, and assured me that I would be all right. I believed this doctor. The staff was wonderful in addressing all my concerns and fear and ensuring I had all the information I needed and my appointments lined up. The staff at the Breast Center always went that extra mile for me. I had a lumpectomy in February 2013, and thankfully the lymph nodes were clear. The course of treatment was radiation therapy.

My support system was great. My husband was my champion, my daughter my caregiver, and my son was my comic relief. And most important . . . my God. In prayer I would always thank God for walking each step of my journey with me, and yes, He carried me at times. My promise to Him was to be an advocate for breast cancer and to help any way I could. I knew the fear and promised Him to help others with the same fear of not knowing what was to come.

Later that year, my company had a major reduction in its workforce, and I was one of them. I took a few months and decided to help at the Breast Center. I would sit in the waiting room with patients and accompany them during the needle localization procedure before breast cancer surgery. I would be there to lend emotional support and hand-holding. I also assisted with the health fairs and assisted with planning and activities with the Johns Hopkins Breast Bayview Medical Center Community Support Group.

I make myself available to newly diagnosed breast cancer patients through friends, co-workers, and just about anyone I meet. I remind women on a monthly basis on Facebook to self-examine, and I stress that early detection is the key to beating this disease. I am an active participant in various breast cancer walks and fundraisers, and my team is known as the "Pink Gorillas." I serve as a strong advocate for breast cancer awareness. Each year I proudly wear a necklace of pink ribbons with names of survivors and those we have lost. The necklace is getting full; too many in my circle of family and friends are being diagnosed with breast cancer. But I am happy to say most are surviving and living life!

My life has changed since the diagnosis. I look at it differently. I'm happier. I cherish my husband, son, daughter, and grandchildren. Life is precious. Fears I had dealt with before breast cancer, I don't have them anymore. I figure if I can beat breast cancer, I can do anything. I'm living life! I'm thankful I wake up each morning. I don't waste time on negativity and I accept the challenge of the unknown. I have come to realize I'm stronger than I thought I was. I do things I would have never thought of doing before my diagnosis. I used to have a fear of flying, which hindered me from seeing the world. Now I fly and have been to Iceland, Alaska, Ireland, Puerto Rico, and many islands in the Caribbean. My next travel experience is Tahiti! I am a survivor!

Felicia Smith

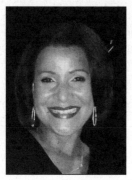

FIGURE 19-3:
Breast cancer survivor Felicia Smith.

Photo used with permission.

Felicia Smith (Figure 19-3) is a field sales representative in the pharmaceutical industry.

At age 47, I was diagnosed with left breast multifocal (two or more areas of cancer) breast cancer in December 2013. I listened to my breast surgeon at Johns Hopkins about the treatment options, length of treatment, and recovery, and I decided to remove both breasts. I knew that my high-paced job and day-to-day commitments, as well as keeping my sanity, wouldn't allow me to entertain the thought of breast cancer coming back, so I had to make a decision that would reduce my risk of recurrence significantly.

I had a mastectomy of the left breast with temporary placement of a tissue expander, until I could complete my final breast reconstruction with my plastic surgeon. I underwent breast reconstruction in August 2014, where my tissue expanders were exchanged with a DIEP flap.

When I look back at my breast cancer experience, I realize why I was diagnosed. I no longer question God. I know that God designed my breast cancer experience to help others and to stop taking life for granted. I continue to be an advocate and navigator for many of my friends and colleagues, supporting them through their breast cancer journeys by connecting them with my breast surgeon and other cancer specialists within Johns Hopkins Bayview Medical Center and Johns Hopkins Hospital. I cannot speak highly enough about my breast surgery team at Johns Hopkins because they helped me to find hope, trust, and the will to live. On the morning of December 11, 2013, my breast surgeon looked me in the eye and told my family members that everything will be okay, and immediately all fear and worry were removed from my mind because he said it with such compassion and sincerity.

Prior to my breast cancer, my life was living on the edge due to the fast pace of my job responsibilities and always having to say yes to things when I should be saying no. Since breast cancer, I've learned to slow down. I have decided to stop and enjoy life. In my personal life, I have committed to being present with my friends, family, and personal relationships. I take time to listen and empathize more, and I am less reactive. I am a mentor for young girls, counseling about the importance of breast exams and screening mammograms.

Life is short, and no one should take it for granted. During my breast cancer journey, I took the time to finalize my living will and testament, ensuring that my beneficiary was listed on all insurance and deed documents. Even though breast cancer didn't take my life, I know that I will die one day. Because of the love I have for my son, I don't want to burden him with planning my funeral. So, yes, I did also plan my funeral. I am celebrating my life to its fullest because I got a second chance of redemption.

At 50, I now look forward to achieving my future goals: retiring sooner, spending more time vacationing, not taking my laptop computer on vacations, and respecting my quiet times.

If I could live through my breast cancer experience again, I would have removed both breasts to avoid me becoming anxious every time I go for a mammogram on the right breast, or worrying whether the right breast will get breast cancer. I am glad that I have my reconstructed breast and my newfound beach abs.

Kelly M.

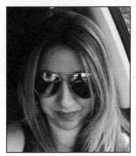

Photo used with permission.

FIGURE 19-4:
Breast cancer survivor Kelly M.

Kelly M. (Figure 19-4) is a criminal investigator who works for the federal government.

At age 37, I was diagnosed with triple negative stage IIB breast cancer in my right breast. I discovered the lump while eight months pregnant with my son. I informed my OB doctor of the strange bump. She believed that it could have been a clogged milk duct as a result of my pregnancy. At my six-week postpartum appointment, my doctor decided it would be a good idea to have the lump checked out. Little did I know, my entire world would change a few days later with one phone call.

I was told the lump was cancerous, and I should see a surgeon right away. In October 2013, following that call, I met with two breast surgeons (from different institutions) who made treatment recommendations for my breast cancer. That's when I met with Dr. Habibi, Dr. Jelovac, and the rest of my amazing breast cancer team at Johns Hopkins Bayview Medical Center. I followed the recommended course of treatment, which included chemotherapy, radiation, and sentinel lymph node dissection with a right lumpectomy over the course of the following year. It was a difficult road as I fought my cancer while taking care of a newborn and a preschooler, all while continuing to work full time at a very demanding job. There were too many times I would just break into tears out of nowhere at any given moment. But my family and friends, especially my babies, kept me going and made me want to fight even harder. My fight with cancer was truly a team effort, and today I stand here almost four years later, stronger and resilient.

When I look back at my breast cancer experience, I realize I should slow things down and take time to stop and smell the roses, as well as not allow myself to get stressed about every obstacle or conflict. Yes, I know it's hard to work 50+ hours per week and be a mother, wife, daughter, and friend. Tomorrow is never promised, and you should live life with that in mind, day in and day out. So I continue to reach out to others diagnosed with breast cancer and other cancers and give them guidance, and even advocate for them as best as I can. Sometimes that means answering questions, offering advice, or just listening. Anyone who faces a cancer diagnosis, whether personally or with a close family member, needs to embrace the fight in their own way, and others should be respectful of their choices. The one piece of advice I would give anyone facing cancer is to take it one day at a time and fight, fight, fight so that one day you can help someone else realize that this, too, shall pass.

I look forward to retiring in about ten years and watching my children fulfill their dreams while my husband continues to drive me crazy as we go through the nesting phase and grow old together.

Joy Walker

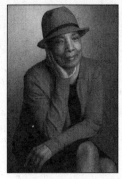

Joy Walker (Figure 19-5) is a rehabilitation counselor. Her sight began failing in her early teens, and she visited the United States from Jamaica, seeking a diagnosis. Declared legally blind, Joy returned to the U.S. as a permanent resident in 1972. After obtaining rehabilitation services for psychosocial adjustment to visual impairment from the Carroll Center for the Blind, in Newton, Massachusetts, she earned a bachelor's degree in rehabilitation counseling from Springfield College, Massachusetts.

Before becoming a stay-at-home mom, Joy worked as a counselor and as a Braille and communication skills instructor with special-needs blind adults at the Therapeutic Living Center for the Blind in Pasadena, California. She homeschooled her two children until divorce and a diagnosis of breast cancer curtailed those efforts.

At age 48, shortly after the divorce and her mother's death, Joy was launched into menopause by the first chemotherapy treatment. This only intensified her struggle as a legally blind single mom raising two teenagers. While enduring 8 rounds of chemotherapy and 36 radiation treatments, Joy attended classes at the Braille Institute in Los Angeles, where she acquired computer skills through the use of adaptive technology. Nine years after her mastectomy, she chose to have reconstructive surgery, which, as she puts it, "made me feel normal again."

In 2016, Joy Walker self-published her book *Journey to Joy: An Inspirational Memoir*, in which she vividly describes her journey with breast cancer, expressing her emotions in spellbinding poetry and prose.

As a 21-year cancer survivor, Joy continues to be an advocate and speaker for various organizations, using her gifts of poetry and music to encourage others. She is known nationally as a writer, poet, musician, and most of all as a breast cancer survivor speaker.

Abbie Savadera

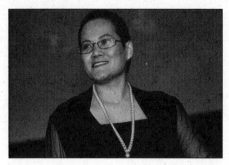

Abbie Savadera (Figure 19-6) is a registered nurse.

Prior to my 46th birthday, I decided to have a very short pixie haircut. I was enjoying my day when I suddenly felt a severe pain on my left leg. I decided to see my doctor for help. I was not given any pain medication, but a multivitamin, and she scheduled me for mammogram, an overdue test. I was relieved from the pain after I took the multivitamins. I ignored my doctor's call until I was done with my summer activities.

It was August 2, 2013, when she broke the news that my mammogram showed a mass on my left breast. I did not accept the mammogram result until I had a left breast ultrasound-guided biopsy of the mass. I was then diagnosed with an invasive ductal carcinoma. I had my left breast mastectomy and sentinel lymph node biopsy in October 2013. I was then confirmed to have stage I left breast–infiltrating ductal carcinoma and was negative for disease in the lymph nodes. I have since been on tamoxifen therapy.

My life changed after the surgery. The journey through breast cancer made me realized that life is too short to waste. With the best team of doctors and nurses, it made my experience lighter and brought me things I hadn't done in my life. I had my first fashion show "Fashion Saves Lives" (sponsored by the American Breast Cancer Foundation) together with the most beautiful breast cancer survivors and had many opportunities to share my breast cancer story. I became an advocate to friends, family, and co-workers about the importance of breast cancer screening and following up with additional testing in a timely manner.

I have made a choice to enjoy my life and to fully trust God. I never questioned God as to why I had to have breast cancer, but instead I asked what it is He wants me to do with cancer. He healed me and He will also heal others too. I will always be grateful for my journey.

Rhonda M. Smith

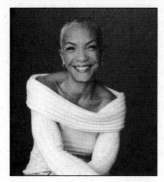

Rhonda M. Smith (Figure 19-7) is an eight-year breast cancer survivor and founder of Breast Cancer Partner (www.breastcancerpartner.com), a for-profit consulting organization with expertise in breast health education and breast cancer disparities, survivorship, and advocacy. She also has experience in developing and implementing community outreach, health promotion, and health behavior change strategies. She currently oversees a women's health initiative focused on heart health, breast health, and diabetes to improve outcomes for underserved women in Alameda and Contra Costa counties in California.

Rhonda is also the Project Director for the Live Healthy OC Initiative, a three-year initiative that aims to transform the model of care from disease-focused to prevention and wellness. She previously served as the consultant/statewide project manager for the Susan G. Komen Circle of Promise California Initiative, an intensive two-year effort to identify evidence-based strategies to decrease the high mortality rate of African American women diagnosed with breast cancer and address disparities at the system, community, and individual levels.

Rhonda has also consulted on an NIH/NCI-funded breast cancer survivorship research study at the Sylvester Comprehensive Cancer Center in Miami, Florida, targeting the diverse population of Black women in the South Florida community. Her responsibilities included marketing, PR, community outreach and recruitment, and facilitating the study's ten-week health and wellness education program to the control group cohorts.

Prior to her breast cancer diagnosis, Rhonda enjoyed a career that expanded more than 25 years of experience in sales, marketing, learning and development consulting, and business management with companies such as Eli Lilly and DuPont. Rhonda has broad international consulting experience and has managed client engagements and projects on 5 continents and in more than 20 countries. Rhonda's international consulting experience includes developing and implementing initiatives for companies such as GE, Office Depot, Johnson & Johnson, Bristol Myers Squibb, Glaxo SmithKline, Abbott Laboratories, Novartis, Rolls Royce, and Xerox Corp.

Rhonda appeared in the October 2010 issue of *More* magazine as a first runner-up in the magazine's essay contest on "Why This Is the Most Fabulous Time in My Life." She wrote an essay about her breast cancer journey and how she has emerged from that experience with a new identity and sense of purpose. Rhonda was also chosen to participate on the 2012 Merz Aesthetics' expert advisory panel for their Stand and Deliver campaign, a national initiative that recognizes women who stand up for causes they believe in and have an impact in their community. Rhonda was also profiled and recognized as a woman who stands and delivers on the *More* magazine *Reinvention* TV show in November 2011.

Rosa Amelia Tena-Krapes

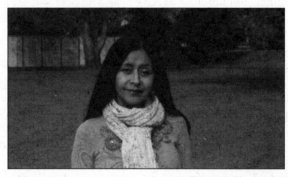

FIGURE 19-8: Breast cancer survivor Rosa Amelia Tena-Krapes.

Photo used with permission.

Rosa Amelia Tena-Krapes (Figure 19-8) is a health educator and advocate dedicated to improving breast cancer awareness and supportive services in Latino communities in the California city of Santa Clarita and surrounding localities.

> My name is Amelia Tena, and I am a twice breast cancer survivor. I work with Valley Care Community Consortium, a nonprofit organization. I lead a collaboration of public and private community partners to advocate, plan, assess needs, and facilitate the development of effective programs and policies to improve the health of the residents in the San Fernando and Santa Clarita valleys.

As a health educator, I work in the Nutrition Education Obesity Prevention Program funded by California Department of Public Health's Network for a Healthy California, with funding from USDA SNAP-ED, known in California as CalFresh, which provides assistance to low-income households to help buy nutritious food for better health.

One of my roles in working with the community in the San Fernando Valley is promoting fitness and good nutrition through weekly series of classes. It also gives me the opportunity to share my story as a breast cancer survivor and bring the awareness into the Latino community, where the resources sometimes are very limited — for reasons including language barriers and cultural competence. I am using my expertise to improve how research studies and clinical care benefit the Latino and medically undeserved communities.

I've volunteered at two Spanish support groups for the past seven years. It's very important to advocate for you and to stay informed of all your options. I share with other cancer patients as a volunteer with the Aliada program at the Cancer Support Community. As an Aliada, I help Spanish-speaking cancer patients navigate the healthcare system and stay informed throughout their cancer journey.

The more knowledge you have, the better control you have as a patient with your health and your emotions.

Linda Butzner

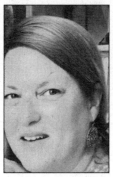

FIGURE 19-9: Breast cancer survivor Linda Butzner.

Photo used with permission.

Linda Butzner (Figure 19-9) is a registered nurse at Wound Care Specialty Center.

My breast cancer was diagnosed during a routine mammogram when I was 47 years old. To say I was shocked is an understatement. To be walking around feeling perfectly healthy and then be told you have a potentially life-threatening illness takes your breath away. From the very beginning, I had no fear — a lot of anxiety for what was to come, but no fear. I had the utmost confidence in my surgical, oncology, and radiation treatment team. I felt sure of the decisions I made, the support I would have from family and friends, and my strong faith in God.

I chose to have a lumpectomy, followed by radiation because my cancer was estrogen-positive. It wasn't easy, and for the first time in my adult life, I had to allow myself to be taken care of — I was used to being the caretaker in my personal and professional lives.

I returned to work as a registered nurse five months after my treatments ended. I quickly found out that I would never be the same physically. I could no longer tolerate the 12-hour shifts and the physical demands of nursing due to the lifelong effects of what I had been through. It took me a year to admit this to myself, but I eventually found a less demanding job in another area of nursing.

Life after breast cancer has changed me in many ways, physically and mentally. The most significant lesson I have convinced myself to embrace is to always choose joy in this life. Don't allow anyone or anything into your life that doesn't bring you happiness. The amount of time we have been given on this earth can't be taken for granted. Wake up every day with a purpose and make a conscious decision to choose joy for yourself.

Alice Loh

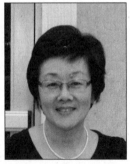

FIGURE 19-10:
Breast cancer survivor Alice Loh.

Photo used with permission.

Alice Loh (Figure 19-10) is currently the breast health project director at Herald Cancer Association (HCA) in San Gabriel, California. Established in 2002, HCA is a nonprofit community organization with the aim of fighting against cancer by (1) raising cancer awareness through public education, (2) increasing the survival rate of cancer patients through early detection and prevention programs, and (3) assisting cancer patients and their families with proper guidance and support groups toward an improved quality of life. HCA also works as a bridge between the portion of the Chinese American community affected by cancer and the entire Chinese American community at large.

As breast health project director, Alice is involved in the planning and implementation of a variety of breast health and breast cancer–related programs, events, and research projects. She has been the lead staff for the breast cancer support program Joy Luck Academy (JLA) since its inception in 2010. JLA is a social support intervention designed to provide both informational and emotional support through two major components: peer mentoring and education. JLA has also been a five-year research project since September 2014.

Alice first became a volunteer at HCA in 2008 after her own encounter with breast cancer and later joined the staff team in 2010. As a breast cancer survivor, she feels a special connection with other women who have been touched by the disease. She is grateful for the opportunity to serve the local Chinese American community with her personal experience. She is also sharing her experience and community expertise by partnering with researchers at City of Hope to bring voice to the Asian community, particularly the Chinese community, in breast cancer research and culturally responsive care.

Alice was born in Taiwan and immigrated to the United States in the early 1970s. She is happily married to her husband of over 35 years, and they have three grown children. Outside of work, she enjoys traveling to foreign countries, experiencing interesting cultures, and tasting delectable cuisines.

Chapter **20**

Ten Ways Family and Friends Can Help You

This chapter offers advice not for you, but for your family and friends, on ways they can help you through your breast cancer experience.

Learn to Listen

Sometimes the most important way a friend or family member can support you throughout your breast cancer diagnosis, treatment, and recovery is *to listen*. Too often everyone wants to give advice when all you really need is someone to listen to you, acknowledge the difficulty of the situation, and learn from your experience.

Another part of learning to listen is for family and friends to refrain from telling you how to feel. No one should be trying to tell you how you should feel because they are not you — they are not walking in your shoes. *You* get to call the shots on how you feel, and all they need to do is listen and acknowledge your feelings.

Be Your Advocate and Note Taker

Being diagnosed with breast cancer and having to coordinate multiple appointments and follow-up visits with your cancer doctors can be mentally overwhelming. It's quite easy to forget details or become confused. Some patients even describe this feeling as going into a "fog." Having a friend or family member come to every appointment with you and take notes while the doctors or nurses discuss your treatments and recovery process is very helpful to you obtaining the best health outcome. Having someone to pay attention to details and stand up for you in terms of sharing the symptoms, side effects, or changes they have observed to your cancer doctor can help you to recover better.

Keep It Lighthearted

Family and friends can keep your spirits up by finding humor and laughter in regular activities or discussions. Laughter, as they say, is good for the soul.

The benefits of laughter are many. Laughter

>> Lowers blood pressure.

>> Reduces stress hormone levels (including cortisol). It helps reduce the anxiety and stress that impact your health and body. Additionally, reduction in stress hormones may result in higher immune system performance.

>> Improves heart health. Laughter gets your heart pumping and burns a similar amount of calories per hour as walking at a slow to moderate pace.

>> Works your abdominal muscles. It helps tone your abs because the muscles in your stomach expand and contract, similar to when you intentionally exercise your abs.

>> Boosts T-cells, specialized immune system cells that when activated fight sickness.

>> Triggers the release of endorphins. Endorphins are great natural painkillers. Therefore laughter can give some relief to chronic pain and make you feel good all over.

>> Produces an overall sense of well-being. Research has shown that people who laugh a lot have a positive outlook on life and fight off diseases quicker than individuals who have a negative outlook on life or who do not laugh as often.

Laughter is a powerful antidote to stress, pain, and conflict. Nothing works faster to bring your mind and body back into balance than a hearty good laugh. Humor lightens your burdens, connects you to others, inspires hopes, and keeps you focused, alert, and grounded. Laughter has the power to heal and renew, and when used frequently it is a tremendous solution for conflicts and problems, enhances your relationships, and supports your physical and emotional health.

Distract You with a Surprise

The gift of distraction from treatment or its side effects can be therapeutic. Friends and families can surprise you with silly gifts, even when it's not your birthday or a major holiday. Thinking about the effort that your loved one took into getting the surprise ready for you lets you know that you are loved and cared for. That is a perfect distraction.

Help You Understand That You Need Help

Sometimes it's difficult to rely on someone else to buy groceries, clean the house, or drop the kids off at school. But your family and friends can be that constant reminder for you that no man is an island, and we need someone, sometimes.

Talk openly and honestly with your loved ones about maximizing your independence, about your physical limitations, about what you are willing to let others do for you, and about ongoing demands you are facing and need to find balance. Make sure your conversations are clear. The importance of asking for help is to say *yes* and accept help from your loved ones. This allows your loved ones to feel connected to you during a time that they really need to express how much they care about you.

Having that person tell you that you must be receptive toward the help they're providing you can be therapeutic for them, too, in dealing with your illness. You need to help people help you.

Leave a Message after the Tone

We often hear family members say that they will call their loved one with breast cancer but don't leave a message on the voicemail because they don't want to be a bother. That's the opposite that they should be doing. There should be no shortage of good wishes. In the lowest moments of despair or discomfort that you may experience from breast cancer treatment, just being able to play back positive messages can make you laugh and feel better overall. The other benefit of friends and family members leaving a message is that you can respond to their messages on your own terms.

Ask You Before Bringing Food

Sometimes you may experience changes in taste or appetite and even energy, or cooking a meal may not be on your agenda. It's great for your family and friends to let you know when they are bringing food so you can have an input on what type of food you may have a taste for and the quantity. This will help you avoid feeling guilty when you're not eating all the food that was given to you.

Buy You Groceries Instead of Bringing Prepared Foods

It would be so cool if your friends came over to your kitchen and took note of what groceries you need or what you would like to eat — and then go buy the groceries. The list may even be typed up and shared via email to other friends and family members, who can all participate in buying your groceries. This ensures that you receive the items you need.

Help Make Life Normal for Your Kids

Your friends and family members can chip in and drive your children to school, football practice, or a friend's birthday party. If the kids are accustomed to going to the grocery store with you, maybe your friends or family members can take them along when they're shopping for your groceries.

Don't Forget You

Part of being human is that when there's a crisis, we tend to rush in to help — but when the immediate crisis is over, everyone is nowhere to be found. The breast cancer journey is long and it may involve side effects from treatment two to three years after, or even five to ten years after initial treatment when receiving hormonal therapy. Even if you don't need family or friends to buy groceries or drive your kids to school, it's nice for them to check in on you from time to time.

Chapter **21**

(At Least) Ten Ways Life Can Be Better After Cancer

Having breast cancer can be a massive wake-up call for anybody. For a start, it makes you wonder what may have caused it. You may start looking at your environment, diet, lifestyle, and stress levels.

Breast cancer survivors often feel a sense of loss and isolation after completing their treatment for breast cancer. Individuals of African and Asian descent and other ethnic minorities often have additional needs because of cultural differences and may feel isolated or have difficulty communicating to others about their health or emotions because they expect that their needs will not be met.

Every breast cancer survivor should get the support they need to live well beyond breast cancer. This chapter offers ten ways your life can be better after breast cancer.

Adopting an Attitude of Gratitude

Your breast cancer experience can teach you how precious life is and that you shouldn't take life for granted. Every day you should stop and smell the roses. Bask yourself in the natural beauty of flowers, trees, skies, fresh air, and the wonders of the human body. Don't let a day go by without having an *attitude of gratitude*. You must remember that there is someone out there going through something worse than you are, whether that's suffering an illness, losing a job, going through a divorce, or grieving for a loved one.

Enjoying the Moment

It doesn't matter if you're 20 or 90, you have things you want to do in your lifetime. We all do. And because you were given a second chance by surviving breast cancer, go ahead and take that leap. You may have always wanted to make that trip to the Grand Canyon, Madagascar, Kenya, the Eiffel Tower in Paris, or even Carnival in Trinidad and Tobago — and now is the time.

REMEMBER

Time wasted never comes around again. Experience something new and enjoy the thrill of stepping outside of your box. One nurse we know wrote a resignation letter to her hospital at the end of her breast cancer treatment, sold her house, and relocated to the Bahamas because she didn't want to continue in a stressful job anymore.

Knowing Why You Deserve Happiness

You may be in an unhealthy or stressful relationship in which you have lost yourself or lost your way. You may have pushed away or taken for granted someone who loves you or wants to be close to you. This is the time when you may reflect on your happiness. Everyone wants to experience happiness at least once in a lifetime, and the time is now. Don't ever think you're unworthy and don't ever feel guilty about wanting to be happy. Don't dwell on your sorrow and stop thinking you're not valuable.

Here are more reasons why you deserve to be happy:

>> **It's your reward for hardship.** You've been through so many rough days, and it's time for you to be rewarded. It's time to balance those bad times with good times. Never assume that life will continue to go downhill — there's always a way back up the hill.

>> **You have given happiness.** There were numerous times when you've done something to make a friend or a stranger smile. You've bought your friends, parents, and relatives gifts, you've attended your friends' concerts, and you've given strangers compliments (or even men or women you've found attractive). You've given happiness to many people, and maybe some of them didn't deserve it. It's time some happiness is given to you.

>> **You've waited for it.** You may have waited to get married to your childhood sweetheart. You may have waited nine months to give birth to each child. Maybe you completed several degrees past high school or waited 11 years for that job promotion. You've been living your life, waiting for happiness, and it's time to go out and find it.

>> **You're a good person.** Really think about the life you've led. Sure, there are some moments you may be embarrassed about, and some days you wish you could forget because of negative experiences. You're still a good person.

>> **You've worked hard.** Unless you're someone like a reality TV star or an heir to a wealthy family, you had to work hard in order to achieve what you have in life. Despite what you think, you haven't spent your life sitting around doing nothing. Life takes work and it doesn't allow you to be useless.

>> **You've searched for happiness.** You've probably tried to find the perfect job, wife or husband, or car or house. Once you realize what you want from life, you go out and work hard towards attaining it. Your reward is due.

>> **You're a survivor.** You woke up this morning and every morning before that. You've faced days where there were huge problems that you had to solve or you had to deal with multiple issues that arose. You made it through terrible fights, stressful jobs, and heartbreaking losses. Those things you endure showed your strength and courage. For all those things you survived, you truly deserve happiness. You're in charge of your situation, and you can make your own happiness *if you choose.*

Learning about Your Health

Throughout your diagnosis and treatment of breast cancer, you've come across many pearls of wisdom that you can take away from your experience. You will have learned the importance of screenings and health promotion activities such as regular physical and wellness exams, screening mammograms, colonoscopies, skin surveillance for abnormal skin changes, glaucoma screening, Pap tests (Pap smears), and so forth.

From this book you've also learned how to eat healthy — which types of foods to avoid and which types of foods you can eat in abundance. You've learned the importance of exercise and increasing physical activity, about meditation and laughter, and about the balance of your mental, physical, spiritual, and emotional well-being. Trust us — it will be hard to go back to your old habits after breast cancer. You'll want the healthier you to burst forth like a baby being born into the world.

Learning to Pick Your Battles

There are two things that are the center of conflicts, problems, and issues. It's important for you to know the difference between the two.

>> **A problem:** Typically refers to a matter or situation that is regarded to be harmful, needs to be dealt with, and has a solution.

>> **An issue:** An important topic or problem for debate or discussion, but you can't solve or change the issue.

Battling every conflict that arises can be detrimental to your health because it raises your body's stress response. When your body experiences high levels of stress, that increases the secretion of cortisol hormone, which is produced by the adrenal gland. High levels of cortisol hormone can increase the PH of the body and inflammation, which makes favorable conditions for diseases to strive.

TIP

Only fight about *problems* because they are truly important. Evaluate the consequences of an argument or a decision. Always consider these questions: *is this worth addressing?* and *will I care about this tomorrow?* Never argue for the sake of arguing.

Here are some more ideas on managing conflict:

>> **Make a plan.** Take a moment to calm down and think through the problem.

>> **Pause for the cause.** Review what your motivation in the conflict is. Ask yourself: *is this really the problem, or is it an issue, or is something else bothering me?*

>> **Don't react immediately.** Walk away from the situation or conflict for several minutes. Calm down and consider what an argument or a specific action will accomplish.

>> **Choose the right time.** Never entertain arguing with someone in public or at the time the problem occurs because clouded judgment can cause words to be exchanged that you may regret. Choose another time or place to address the problem when the environment is not threatening and the individuals can be calm.

>> **Talk, never yell.** If your conversation erupts into a yelling match, then both individuals will likely become defensive, and it will end in emotional turmoil.

>> **Agree to disagree.** Compromise is the best solution to solving any conflict. Always stay positive and try to defuse the situation with humor and laughter whenever possible.

>> **Communicate.** Don't assume the other individual knows what you are thinking or feeling. Be specific about communicating what upsets you.

>> **Preempt the problem.** Try to be proactive rather than reactive. Address the situation as soon as you see that a problem will arise.

>> **Discuss the problem in person.** Disagreements are best addressed face to face. Body language and facial expressions help convey your meaning. The other person will know if you are truly sorry, or even if you're truthful. Emails, tweets, and phone conversations can be misinterpreted and may extend the conflict unnecessarily.

Learning to Be in the Here and Now

There is no room for procrastination. You must have a great appreciation for time and know that tomorrow is never promised. Take care of what you can do today because you don't want to add today's list to tomorrow surprises. When you have a list of stuff that should have been done several days ago, it lays an emotional burden on you that often erupts into anxiety, fear, and even depression. Avoid situations that can affect your overall health and well-being. Know that you've got to set realistic goals to ensure that they can be achieved in the time frame that you have set.

Engaging in Positive Self-Talk and Conversations

Positive self-talk is the stuff that makes you feel good about yourself and the things going on in your life. It is like having an optimistic voice in your head that always looks at the cup as half full instead of half empty. You should learn to positively self-talk as you cope through your treatment and look forward to recovering from surgery or chemotherapy. You may have found yourself saying, "It's tough, but I can do this."

This is the mind-over-matter phenomenon. The human spirit is tenacious when you push through using your mental toughness, spirituality, and human connectedness to get through the cancer battle. The human mind and spirit are ultimately more powerful than the human body.

Managing Physical Changes

You may find that you're still coping with the effects of breast treatment on your body. It takes time to get over these effects. You may wonder how your body should feel during this time and what the signs that cancer is coming back are. Many effects from breast cancer treatment can be managed, but you've got to let your doctor know the symptoms you're experiencing. See Table 21-1.

TABLE 21-1   **Common Physical Changes after Breast Cancer Treatment with Possible Solutions**

Physical Changes	Possible Solutions
Cancer-related fatigue	Exercise, small well-balanced meals, structured activities when you have most energy, diet high in iron, referral to hematologist for management of anemia or iron deficiency. Referral to occupational therapist to assist with activities of daily living.
Lack of memory and concentration changes	Referral to neurologist to evaluate memory changes, for mind exercises, and for coping strategies.
Pain	Referral for physical therapy or physical medicine rehabilitation specialist/physiatrist. Referral for radiation or referral to other specialist according to the cause of the pain.
Nervous system changes (neuropathy)	Referral to neurologist or pain specialist to manage the neuropathy or *neuropathic* pain caused by disease or injury to the area in that processes sensory input from the skin, muscles, and joints of the nervous system.
Lymphedema or swelling	Referred to physical therapy/lymphedema specialist.
Mouth or teeth problems	Referral to dentist or dental surgeon.
Changes in weight and eating habits	Referral to nutritionist, personal trainer, GYM or fitness center, and so on.
Trouble swallowing	Referral to speech and language pathologist.
Bladder or bowel control problems	Referral to urologist and pelvic floor rehabilitation specialist.
Menopause symptoms	Referral to gynecologist or endocrinologist.
Mood changes (anxiety, scanxiety, depression)	Referral to psychiatrist, psychologist, or counselor

REMEMBER

Here are some more things to consider:

>> Talk to your doctor about your physical symptoms or side effects from treatment.

>> Schedule your appointment with referred specialist to manage your physical symptoms.

>> Complete all recommended visits and treatment by your specialist to have the best success.

>> In all you do, maintain a healthy diet and healthy mind — and exercise.

Achieving Self-Acceptance and the New You

It's true that positive body image is hard enough in today's world, but having breast cancer treatment can make it even harder. Among the many concerns you may have after breast cancer treatment is the emotional impact of the change in your body. Body image can be defined as what you think of your physical self and how you think others see your body. The loss of or changes to your breasts, hair, physical strength, and/or libido can affect your femininity or masculinity because looks are often equated to sexy or handsome in society. Even when there are no obvious physical changes from breast cancer treatment, body image may still be a concern for the survivor.

TIP

Here are some tips on accepting the new you:

>> Give yourself time to grieve the loss of your breasts, hair, or physical ability before you decide what to do next.

>> Wear clothing that makes you feel comfortable. If you like to wear T-string underwear, continue. If you like to wear shorts, do so.

>> Find clothing that your significant other likes to see you in or that you like to see yourself wear. Don't feel guilty if you feel like covering up a bit more during intimacy until you feel comfortable being naked again. Find new pleasures during intimacy that can incorporate the change in your body.

>> Take advantage of getting the "full works" of breast reconstruction. Consider nipple construction, 3D nipple areolar or areola tattoos, and fat grafting to ensure that the breast looks similar to your normal breast. This will mean going back several times to your plastic surgeon for a little "nipping and tucking."

>> Eat healthy balanced meals and limit alcohol. A good diet can often help you maintain your ideal weight and make you feel physically and emotionally alive and healthy. If you need help, have your doctor refer you to a nutritionist or dietitian.

>> If you have a significant other, talk to them about how you feel. Open communication is the best way to reduce anxiety and discomfort in a relationship. Talk to each other and be open and honest about sex and how you can both find new ways to satisfy each other.

>> If you're single or dating casually, don' be in a rush to "get laid." Take as much time as you need to start a physical relationship. Even though whom you choose to share your body with is your decision, you must be mindful of when a relationship is meaningful or when it is casual. You don't want to get yourself in a vulnerable position wondering if your partner is committed to you. Take your time and find the right person who loves you for you with unconditional love.

>> Seek out professional counseling or therapy if you need a little help with coping with the new you and developing positive self-talk.

Following a Cancer Survivorship Plan

In 2006, the Institute of Medicine issued a report recommending that every cancer patient receive a survivorship care plan from their cancer doctor that includes guidelines for monitoring and maintaining their health.

The plan should include:

>> A written treatment summary, including drug names and dosages, as well as radiation dose, if applicable.

>> An individual follow-up plan.

>> Recommendations about which provider — oncologist, primary care doctor, or other specialist — should be in charge of cancer-related and other medical care.

The best part of this plan is the individual follow-up plan which dictates how often you will follow up with your medical oncologist, radiation oncologist, breast surgeon, primary care provider, and other specialists related to your active conditions. A surveillance summary is usually included to ensure that all your cancer screenings are up to date.

Check out the free downloadable breast cancer survivorship care plan at www.dummies.com. Just search for *detecting and living with breast cancer.*

Screening for Breast Cancer and Wellness

After breast cancer treatment, you may continue to visit your cancer doctor for some time and then transfer your care to a primary care doctor. Screening for recurrence is based on your age, specific diagnosis, and the treatments you received.

In general, the following screening tests and schedules are recommended:

>> **Medical history and physical examination:** Visit your doctor every 3–6 months for the first three years after the first treatment, every 6–12 months for the next two years, and then once each year thereafter.

>> **Mammography:** Schedule a diagnostic mammogram one year after the first mammogram that led to your diagnosis. However, if you have had radiation therapy, wait six months after your last treatment. After this first post-treatment mammogram, mammography is recommended at least every year, either on one or both breasts depending on the type of surgery you received.

>> **Breast self-examination:** Perform a breast self-examination at least every month. This procedure is not a substitute for a mammogram.

>> **Breast MRI:** Schedule your breast MRI every year, six months in between the mammogram if you were determined to be at high risk for breast cancer recurrence or have a 20 percent risk or more of developing breast cancer.

REMEMBER

MRI criteria is evolving quickly. What is recommended now will quickly change in the future. MRI indications are an ongoing topic of debate for clinicians and researchers because there are no firm guidelines. Ask your doctor if you need to have a breast MRI in addition to or instead of a mammogram, especially to look for recurrent breast cancer.

>> **Genetic counseling:** Another important part of follow-up care is to tell your doctor if you have a history of cancer in your family because you may benefit from genetic counseling and testing.

>> **Hormonal therapy:** If it's part of your treatment plan, continue hormonal therapy as directed by your cancer doctor.

And here are wellness screening recommendations:

>> **GYN exam:** Schedule your gynecology exam every year or per screening guidelines every two to three years if you had two consecutive negative Pap smears. However, if you are on hormonal therapy with Tamoxifen, you must have a Pap smear annually.

>> **Physical exam/wellness exam:** Schedule a physical exam or wellness exam yearly. At this exam a comprehensive medical history, physical exam, psychosocial history, evaluation of medications, active symptoms, and comprehensive blood tests will be completed. This type of exam is essential for finding out changes with your body even before symptoms may occur.

>> **Colonoscopy:** Schedule a colonoscopy for colon cancer screening from age 50. If you have a strong family history of colon cancer, talk to your doctor about starting screening at an earlier age.

>> **Prostate cancer screening (for men):** Men should start having prostate cancer screening annually from age 50, including a digital rectal exam (DRE), PSA blood tests, and self-report of urinary symptoms. For men of African descent, prostate cancer screening should start at age 40, due to the increased incidence and mortality in this population. Prostate cancer screening guidelines are controversial, but it is important for you to know your risk and your family risk and to talk to your doctor about the best age for you to start prostate cancer screening.

>> **Dermatology screening:** Schedule skin surveillance for examination of skin lesions or skin changes with a dermatologist every year. This is a sure way to detect skin cancers at an early stage.

>> **Ophthalmology screening (eye exam):** Schedule an eye exam annually or according to guidelines to screen for glaucoma, cataract, or other eye conditions. If you have diabetes and or hypertension, you should be screened every year by an ophthalmologist — a specialist who will dilate your eyes and inspect the retinas and other structures in your eye.

Women and men recovering from breast cancer are encouraged to follow established guidelines for good health, such as reaching and maintaining a healthy weight, exercising, not smoking, eating a balanced diet rich in fruits and vegetables, avoiding concentrated sweets and excessive carbohydrates, and following cancer screening and wellness recommendations.

Appendix A

Breast Health Glossary

This breast health glossary provides brief definitions for many of the terms used throughout the book. You can use this as a quick reference to understanding the words as they relate to the field of breast cancer awareness, diagnosis, treatment, recovery, and survivorship. Some of the definitions come from the website of the National Cancer Institute (www.cancer.gov), which are in the public domain, and some come from the American Breast Cancer Foundation and are used with permission (www.abcf.org).

The American Breast Cancer Foundation (ABCF) is a national 501(c)(3) charity providing educational resources and vital funding to aid in the early detection, treatment, and survival of breast cancer for underserved and uninsured individuals, regardless of age or gender. ABCF addresses many issues and provides resources for many subjects that are addressed in this book.

Adjuvant therapy: Additional cancer treatment given after the primary treatment to reduce the risk that the cancer will come back. Adjuvant therapy may include chemotherapy, radiation therapy, hormone therapy, targeted therapy, or biological therapy.

Anxiety: Feelings of fear, dread, and uneasiness that may occur as a reaction to stress. A person with anxiety may sweat, feel restless and tense, and have a rapid heartbeat. Extreme anxiety that happens often over time may be a sign of an anxiety disorder.

Areola: The area of dark-colored skin on the breast that surrounds the nipple.

Axillary lymph node dissection: Surgery to remove lymph nodes found in the armpit region. Also called axillary dissection.

Axillary node: Any of the lymph nodes of the axilla (underarm); also called axillary glands.

B-cell: A type of white blood cell that makes antibodies. B-cells are part of the immune system and develop from stem cells in the bone marrow. Also called B lymphocyte.

Benign: A mild type that does not threaten health or life; not cancerous.

Biological therapy: A type of treatment that uses substances made from living organisms to treat disease. These substances may occur naturally in the body or may be made in the laboratory. Some biological therapies stimulate or suppress the immune system to help the body fight cancer, infection, and other diseases. Other biological therapies attack specific cancer cells, which may help keep them from growing or kill them. They may also lessen certain side effects caused by some cancer treatments. Types of biological therapy include immunotherapy (such as vaccines, cytokines, and some antibodies), gene therapy, and some targeted therapies. Also called biological response modifier therapy, biotherapy, and BRM therapy.

Biopsy: The removal and examination of tissue or fluid from a living body.

Bloodstream: The flowing blood in a circulatory system.

Brachytherapy (internal radiation): Radiation in which the source is placed.

BRCA1: A gene on chromosome 17 that normally helps to suppress cell growth. A person who inherits certain mutations (changes) in a BRCA1 gene has a higher risk of getting breast, ovarian, prostate, and other types of cancer.

BRCA2: A gene on chromosome 13 that normally helps to suppress cell growth. A person who inherits certain mutations (changes) in a BRCA2 gene has a higher risk of getting breast, ovarian, prostate, and other types of cancer.

Breast cancer: Cancer that originates from the cells of the breast.

Breast density: A term used to describe the amount of dense tissue compared to the amount of fatty tissue in the breast on a mammogram. Dense breast tissue has more fibrous and glandular tissue than fat. There are different levels of breast density, ranging from little or no dense tissue to very dense tissue. The more density, the harder it may be to find tumors or other changes on a mammogram.

Breast-conserving surgery: A mastectomy where only part of the breast containing breast cancer is removed.

Calcification: Abnormal deposits of calcium salts within tissue.

Cancer: A malignant tumor with potentially unlimited growth, that expands locally by invasion and systematically by metastasis.

Cell: The basic building block of life that forms the smallest structural unit of living matter capable of functioning independently.

Chemotherapy: The use of chemical agents in the treatment or control of a disease.

Clinical trial: A type of research study that tests how well new medical approaches work in people. These studies test new methods of screening, prevention, diagnosis, or treatment of a disease. Also called clinical study.

Core needle biopsy: The removal of a tissue sample with a wide needle for examination under a microscope. Also called core biopsy.

Deoxyribonucleic acid (DNA): Any of various nucleic acids that are usually the molecular basis of heredity, are constructed of a double helix held together by hydrogen bonds, and that in eukaryotes are localized mainly in the cell nuclei.

Depression: A mental condition marked by ongoing feelings of sadness, despair, loss of energy, and difficulty dealing with normal daily life. Other symptoms of depression include feelings of worthlessness and hopelessness, loss of pleasure in activities, changes in eating or sleeping habits, and thoughts of death or suicide. Depression can affect anyone and can be successfully treated. Depression affects 15–25 percent of cancer patients.

Diagnosis: The act of identifying a disease from its signs and symptoms.

Diagnostic mammogram: An X-ray image of the breast after an abnormality has been detected.

DIEP flap: A type of breast reconstruction in which blood vessels called deep inferior epigastric perforators (DIEP) and the skin and fat connected to them are removed from the lower abdomen and used for reconstruction. Muscle is left in place.

Diethylstilbestrol (DES): A crystalline synthetic compound used as a potent estrogen that may cause cancer or birth defects in the children of pregnant women.

Distress: Emotional, social, spiritual, or physical pain or suffering that may cause a person to feel sad, afraid, depressed, anxious, or lonely. People in distress may also feel that they are not able to manage or cope with changes caused by normal life activities or by having a disease, such as cancer. Cancer patients may have trouble coping with their diagnosis, physical symptoms, or treatment.

Duct: A bodily tube or vessel that carries the secretion of a gland.

Ductal carcinoma in situ (DCIS): Abnormal cells found in the lining of the breast duct.

Endocrine therapy: Treatment that adds, blocks, or removes hormones. For certain conditions (such as diabetes or menopause), hormones are given to adjust low hormone levels. To slow or stop the growth of certain cancers (such as prostate and breast cancer), synthetic hormones or other drugs may be given to block the body's natural hormones. Sometimes surgery is needed to remove the gland that makes a certain hormone. Also called hormonal therapy, hormone therapy, and hormone treatment.

Estrogen: A natural steroid that stimulates the development of female sex characteristics and promote the growth and maintenance of the female reproductive system.

Estrogen-receptor-positive: Describes cells that have a receptor protein that binds the hormone estrogen. Cancer cells that are estrogen-receptor-positive may need estrogen to grow, and may stop growing or die when treated with substances that block the binding and actions of estrogen. Also called ER+.

External beam radiation: Radiation comes from a machine outside of the body and focuses on the area that has cancer.

Fibroadenoma: Solid, benign breast tumors that often occur in women between the ages of 20–30 years old.

Gene mutation: Mutation or change due to the reorganization of a gene.

Grading: A system for classifying cancer cells in terms of how abnormal they appear when examined under a microscope. The objective of a grading system is to provide information about the probable growth rate of the tumor and its tendency to spread. The systems used to grade tumors vary with each type of cancer. Grading plays a role in treatment decisions.

Heparin: A substance that slows the formation of blood clots. Heparin is made by the liver, lungs, and other tissues in the body and can also be made in the laboratory. Heparin may be injected into muscle or blood to prevent or break up blood clots. It is a type of anticoagulant.

HER2/neu: A protein involved in normal cell growth. It is found on some types of cancer cells, including breast and ovarian. Cancer cells removed from the body may be tested for the presence of HER2/neu to help decide the best type of treatment. HER2/neu is a type of receptor tyrosine kinase. Also called c-erbB-2, human EGF receptor 2, and human epidermal growth factor receptor 2.

HER2/neu test: A laboratory test that measures the amount of HER2/neu protein on cancer cells or how many copies of the HER2 gene are in the DNA. The HER2/neu protein is involved in normal cell growth. It may be made in larger than normal amounts by some types of cancer, including breast, ovarian, bladder, pancreatic, and stomach cancer. This may cause cancer cells to grow more quickly and spread to other parts of the body. A HER2/neu test may be done to help plan treatment. It is a type of tumor marker test. Also called HER2 test and human epidermal growth factor receptor 2 test.

HER2+: Describes cancer cells that have too much of a protein called HER2 on their surface. In normal cells, HER2 helps to control cell growth. When it is made in larger than normal amounts by cancer cells, the cells may grow more quickly and be more likely to spread to other parts of the body. Checking to see if a cancer is HER2+ may help plan treatment, which may include drugs that kill HER2+ cancer cells. Cancers that may be HER2+ include breast, bladder, pancreatic, ovarian, and stomach cancers. Also called c-erbB-2 positive and human epidermal growth factor receptor 2 positive.

Hereditary: Genetically passed from parent to biological child.

Hormonal therapy: Treatment that adds, blocks, or removes hormones. For certain conditions (such as diabetes or menopause), hormones are given to adjust low hormone levels. To slow or stop the growth of certain cancers (such as prostate and breast cancer), synthetic hormones or other drugs may be given to block the body's natural hormones. Sometimes surgery is needed to remove the gland that makes a certain hormone. Also called endocrine therapy, hormone therapy, and hormone treatment.

Hormone-replacement therapy (HRT): An administration of estrogen and synthetic progestin to treat the symptoms of menopause and reduce the risk of postmenopausal osteoporosis.

Infertility: The inability to produce children.

Infiltrating ductal carcinoma (IDC): See invasive ductal carcinoma.

Infiltrating lobular carcinoma (ILC): See invasive lobular carcinoma.

Inflammatory breast cancer: Breast cancer that mainly affects the skin of the breasts.

Infraclavicular nodes: Lymph nodes below the clavicle.

Internal mammary nodes: Lymph nodes in the chest.

Intraductal breast papilloma: A benign (not cancer), wart-like growth in a milk duct of the breast. It is usually found close to the nipple and may cause a discharge from the nipple. It may also cause pain and a lump in the breast that can be felt. It usually affects women aged 35–55 years. Having a single papilloma does not increase the risk of breast cancer. When there are multiple intraductal breast papillomas, they are usually found farther from the nipple. There may not be a nipple discharge and the papillomas may not be felt. Having multiple intraductal breast papillomas may increase the risk of breast cancer. Also called intraductal papilloma.

Intraductal carcinoma: Another name for ductal carcinoma in situ (DCIS); a non invasive breast cancer in which abnormal cells have not spread through the ducts into surrounding breast tissue.

Invasive: Tending to spread and invade healthy tissue.

Invasive ductal carcinoma (IDC): Breast cancer that has started in the ducts of the breasts and can invade tissue surrounding the ducts.

Invasive lobular carcinoma (ILC): Breast cancer that has started in the lobules of the breast and can invade other parts of the body.

Killer T-cell: A type of immune cell that can kill certain cells, including foreign cells, cancer cells, and cells infected with a virus. Killer T-cells can be separated from other blood cells, grown in the laboratory, and then given to a patient to kill cancer cells. A killer T-cell is a type of white blood cell and a type of lymphocyte. Also called cytotoxic T-cell and cytotoxic T lymphocyte.

Lobular carcinoma in situ (LCIS): Abnormal cells that are found in the lobules of the breast.

Lobular neoplasia: Another name for lobular carcinoma in situ (LCIS); abnormal cell growth appears in the lobules of the breast, not a true cancer due to the unlikelihood of it spreading to surrounding tissues.

Lobule: Glands in the breasts that produce milk.

Lymph: Fluid that contains tissue, waste products, and immune cells.

Lymph nodes: Small clusters of immune system cells that help fight infection.

Lymph system: Part of the circulatory system that scavenges fluids and proteins that have escaped from cells and tissues and returns them to the blood.

Lymphatic vessels: Tubes that carry clear fluid called lymph away from the breast.

Macrocalcification: A small deposit of calcium in the breast.

Male breast cancer: A rare form of cancer that occurs in the breasts of a male.

Malignant: Tending to metastasize, and terminate fatally; the opposite of benign.

MammaPrint: A test that is used to help predict whether breast cancer has spread to other parts of the body or come back. The test looks at the activity of 70 different genes in breast cancer tissue of women who have early-stage breast cancer that has not spread to the lymph nodes. If there is a high risk that the cancer will spread or come back, it may be used to help plan treatment with anticancer drugs. Also called 70-gene signature.

Mammogram: An X-ray image of the breast.

Mantle radiation: The area of the neck, chest, and lymph nodes in the armpit that are exposed to radiation therapy.

Mastectomy: A procedure in which the breast tissue, and possibly some surrounding tissue is removed.

Metastasis: The spread of cancer cells from the initial site of disease to another part of the body.

Metastatic breast cancer: Breast cancer that has invaded other parts of the body outside of the breasts.

Microcalcification: A tiny deposit of calcium in the breast.

Modified radical mastectomy: A simple mastectomy with the removal of underarm lymph nodes.

MRI: A procedure in which radio waves and a powerful magnet linked to a computer are used to create detailed pictures of areas inside the body. These pictures can show the difference between normal and diseased tissue. MRI makes better images of organs and soft tissue than other scanning techniques, such as computed tomography (CT) or X-ray. MRI is especially useful for imaging the brain, the spine, the soft tissue of joints, and the inside of bones. Also called magnetic resonance imaging, NMRI, and nuclear magnetic resonance imaging.

Mutation: A permanent change in hereditary material.

Needle aspiration: The process of obtaining a sample of cells and bits of tissue for examination by suctioning through a needle attached to a syringe.

Neoadjuvant therapy: Treatment given as a first step to shrink a tumor before the main treatment, which is usually surgery, is given. Examples of neoadjuvant therapy include chemotherapy, radiation therapy, and hormone therapy. It is a type of induction therapy.

Nipple retraction: When the nipple turns inwards.

Noninvasive: In medicine, it describes a procedure that does not require inserting an instrument through the skin or into a body opening. In cancer, it describes a disease that has not spread outside the tissue in which it began.

Oncotype DX: A test that is used to help predict whether breast cancer will spread to other parts of the body or come back. The test looks at the activity of 21 different genes in breast cancer tissue of women who have early-stage breast cancer that is estrogen-receptor-positive and has not spread to the lymph nodes. If there is a high risk that the cancer will spread or come back, it may be used to help plan treatment with anti-cancer drugs. Also called 21-gene signature.

Organ: A structure consisting of cells and tissues that can perform a specific function in an organism.

Paget's disease: Abnormal cells found in the lining of the breast duct.

Pathology report: The description of cells and tissues made by a pathologist based on microscopic evidence, and sometimes used to make a diagnosis of a disease.

Precancerous: A term used to describe a condition that may (or is likely to) become cancer. Also called premalignant.

Precision medicine: A form of medicine that uses information about a person's genes, proteins, and environment to prevent, diagnose, and treat disease. In cancer, precision medicine uses specific information about a person's tumor to help diagnose, plan treatment, find out how well treatment is working, or make a prognosis. Examples of precision medicine include using targeted therapies to treat specific types of cancer cells, such as HER2+ breast cancer cells, or using tumor marker testing to help diagnose cancer. Also called personalized medicine.

Pre-operative: Care given in preparation for surgery that may include lab tests being drawn, imaging tests, and a physical exam.

Progesterone: A hormone that occurs naturally in women.

Prognosis: A doctor's opinion about how an individual will recover from an illness or injury.

Prolactin: A hormone that is made by the pituitary gland (a pea-sized organ in the center of the brain). Prolactin causes a woman's breasts to make milk during and after pregnancy and has many other effects in the body.

Prophylactic mastectomy: Surgery to reduce the risk of developing breast cancer by removing one or both breasts before disease develops. Also called preventive mastectomy.

Protective factor: Habits or behaviors that can reduce your risk of developing a disease and improve your overall health.

Protein-receptor: A molecule inside or on the surface of a cell (that is made of protein) that binds to a specific substance and causes a specific effect in the cell.

Radiation: Energy radiated in the form of waves or particles.

Radical mastectomy: Removal of the entire breast, underarm lymph nodes, and chest wall muscles under the breast.

Radiologist: A doctor who specializes in the use of radiant energy for diagnostic and therapeutic purposes.

Receptor-positive: Specific protein receptors that are found on the surface of a cell and may be in large quantities.

Reconstructive surgery: A procedure done to restore the appearance of the breast after a mastectomy or breast-conserving surgery.

Risk factor: Something that increases the chance of developing a disease. Some examples of risk factors for cancer are age, a family history of certain cancers, use of tobacco products, being exposed to radiation or certain chemicals, infection with certain viruses or bacteria, and certain genetic changes.

Screening mammogram: An X-ray image of the breast taken before an abnormality is detected.

Sentinel lymph node: The first lymph node that cancer cells go to from the primary tumor.

Sentinel lymph node biopsy (SLNB): A procedure that may be used to determine if one or more lymph nodes contain cancer cells.

Sexuality: A person's behaviors, desires, and attitudes related to sex and physical intimacy with others.

Side effect: A secondary and usually adverse effect of a drug.

Simple cyst: A fluid-filled benign sac found in the breast.

Simple mastectomy: A mastectomy in which the entire breast is removed, including the nipple.

Skin-sparing mastectomy: A mastectomy where most of the skin over the breast, not including the nipple or areola, is left intact.

Sleep apnea: A sleep disorder that is marked by pauses in breathing of 10 seconds or more during sleep, and causes unrestful sleep. Symptoms include loud or abnormal snoring, daytime sleepiness, irritability, and depression.

Stage 0 breast carcinoma in situ: There are three types of stage 0 breast carcinoma in situ: ductal carcinoma in situ (DCIS), lobular carcinoma in situ (LCIS), and Paget's disease of the nipple. DCIS is a noninvasive condition in which abnormal cells are found in the lining of a breast duct. The abnormal cells have not spread outside the duct to other tissues in the breast. In some cases, DCIS may become invasive cancer and spread to other tissues. At this time, there is no way to know which lesions could become invasive. LCIS is a condition in which abnormal cells are found in the lobules of the breast. This condition seldom becomes invasive cancer. However, having LCIS in one breast increases the risk of developing breast cancer in either breast. Paget's disease of the nipple is a condition in which abnormal cells are found in the nipple only. Also called breast carcinoma in situ.

Stage I breast cancer: Stage I is divided into stages IA and IB. In stage IA, the tumor is 2 centimeters or smaller. Cancer has not spread outside the breast. In stage IB, small clusters of breast cancer cells (larger than 0.2 millimeter but not larger than 2 millimeters) are found in the lymph nodes and either: (1) no tumor is found in the breast; or (2) the tumor is 2 centimeters or smaller.

Stage II breast cancer: Stage II is divided into stages IIA and IIB. In stage IIA, (1) no tumor is found in the breast or the tumor is 2 centimeters or smaller. Cancer (larger than 2 millimeters) is found in one to three axillary lymph nodes or in the lymph nodes near the breastbone (found during a sentinel lymph node biopsy); or (2) the tumor is larger than 2 centimeters but not larger than 5 centimeters. Cancer has not spread to the lymph nodes. In stage IIB, the tumor is (1) larger than 2 centimeters but not larger than 5 centimeters. Small clusters of breast cancer cells (larger than 0.2 millimeter but not larger than 2 millimeters) are found in the lymph nodes; or (2) larger than 2 centimeters but not larger than 5 centimeters. Cancer has spread to one to three axillary lymph nodes or to the lymph nodes near the breastbone (found during a sentinel lymph node biopsy); or (3) larger than 5 centimeters. Cancer has not spread to the lymph nodes.

Stage III breast cancer: Stage III is divided into stages IIIA, IIIB, and IIIC. In stage IIIA, (1) no tumor is found in the breast or the tumor may be any size. Cancer is found in four to nine axillary lymph nodes or in the lymph nodes near the breastbone (found during imaging tests or a physical exam); or (2) the tumor is larger than 5 centimeters. Small clusters of breast cancer cells (larger than 0.2 millimeter but not larger than 2 millimeters) are found in the lymph nodes; or (3) the tumor is larger than 5 centimeters. Cancer has spread to one to three axillary lymph nodes or to the lymph nodes near the breastbone (found during a sentinel lymph node biopsy). In stage IIIB, the tumor may be any size and cancer has spread to the chest wall and/or to the skin of the breast and caused swelling or an ulcer. Also, cancer may have spread to: (1) up to nine axillary lymph nodes; or (2) the lymph nodes near the breastbone. Cancer that has spread to the skin of the breast may also be inflammatory breast cancer. In stage IIIC, no tumor is found in the breast or the tumor may be any size. Cancer may have spread to the skin of the breast and caused swelling or an ulcer and/or has spread to the chest wall. Also, cancer has spread to: (1) 10 or more axillary lymph nodes; or (2) lymph nodes above or below the collarbone; or (3) axillary lymph nodes and lymph nodes near the breastbone. Cancer that has spread to the skin of the breast may also be inflammatory breast cancer. For treatment, stage IIIC breast cancer is divided into operable and inoperable stage IIIC.

Stage IV breast cancer: Cancer has spread to other organs of the body, most often the bones, lungs, liver, or brain.

Staging: Performing exams and tests to learn the extent of the cancer within the body, especially whether the disease has spread from the original site to other parts of the body. It is important to know the stage of the disease in order to plan the best treatment.

Staging system: A system that is used to describe the extent of cancer in the body. Staging is usually based on the size of the tumor and whether the cancer has spread from where it started to nearby areas, lymph nodes, or other parts of the body.

Stereotactic biopsy: A biopsy procedure that uses a computer and a 3D scanning device to find a tumor site and guide the removal of tissue for examination under a microscope.

Stroma: Connective and fatty tissue that makes up the breast and encompasses the ducts, lobules, blood vessels, and lymphatic vessels.

Support group: A group of people with similar disease or concerns who help each other cope by sharing experiences and information.

Supraclavicular nodes: Lymph nodes located above the clavicle.

Survivorship: In cancer, survivorship focuses on the health and life of a person with cancer post treatment until the end of life. It covers the physical, psychosocial, and economic issues of cancer, beyond the diagnosis and treatment phases. Survivorship includes issues related to the ability to get healthcare and follow-up treatment, late effects of treatment, second cancers, and quality of life. Family members, friends, and caregivers are also considered part of the survivorship experience.

Survivorship care plan: A detailed plan for a patient's follow-up care after treatment for a disease ends. In cancer, the plan is based on the type of cancer and the treatment the patient received. A survivorship care plan may include schedules for physical exams and medical tests to see if the cancer has come back or spread to other parts of the body. Follow-up care also checks for health problems that may occur months or years after treatment ends, including other types of cancer. A survivorship care plan may also include information to help meet the emotional, social, legal, and financial needs of the patient. It may include referrals to specialists and recommendations for a healthy lifestyle, such as changes in diet and exercise and quitting smoking. Also called follow-up care plan.

TIP

You can find a free downloadable survivorship care plan on www.dummies.com — just search for *detecting and living with breast cancer.*

Symptom: Something that indicates evidence of possible disease or physical disturbance.

T-cell: A type of white blood cell. T-cells are part of the immune system and develop from stem cells in the bone marrow. They help protect the body from infection and may help fight cancer. Also called T lymphocyte and thymocyte.

Tamoxifen: A drug used to treat certain types of breast cancer in women and men. It is also used to prevent breast cancer in women who have had ductal carcinoma in situ (abnormal cells in the ducts of the breast) and in women who are at a high risk of developing breast cancer. Tamoxifen is also being studied in the treatment of other types of cancer. It blocks the effects of the hormone estrogen in the breast. Tamoxifen is a type of antiestrogen. Also called tamoxifen citrate.

Targeted therapy: A type of treatment that uses drugs or other substances to identify and attack specific types of cancer cells with less harm to normal cells. Some targeted therapies block the action of certain enzymes, proteins, or other molecules involved in the growth and spread of cancer cells. Other types of targeted therapies help the immune system kill cancer cells or deliver toxic substances directly to cancer cells and kill them. Targeted therapy may have fewer side effects than other types of cancer treatment. Most targeted therapies are either small molecule drugs or monoclonal antibodies.

Tissue: A collection of cells of a particular kind that forms one of the structural materials of an animal.

TNM staging system: A system to describe the amount and spread of cancer in a patient's body, using TNM. T describes the size of the tumor and any spread of cancer into nearby tissue; N describes spread of cancer to nearby lymph nodes; and M describes metastasis (spread of cancer to other parts of the body). This system was created and is updated by the American Joint Committee on Cancer (AJCC) and the International Union Against Cancer (UICC). The TNM staging system is used to describe most types of cancer. Also called AJCC staging system.

Triple-negative breast cancer: Breast cancer in which cells do not have genes for the following receptors: progesterone, estrogen, and HER2/neu (human epidermal growth receptor 2).

Tumor: A solid, abnormal new growth of tissue that arises from rapid cell growth.

Ultrasound (sonography): A noninvasive technique that uses sound waves to examine internal body structures.

Appendix B

Support Groups, Resources, and Organizations

There are many local, regional, and international support groups or support networks for breast cancer survivors. Collectively, the main goal of support groups is to deliver emotional, physical, or financial support by providing resources to assist the breast cancer survivor throughout treatment and beyond.

Support groups may be organized at the grassroots level, where a cancer survivor or a community advocate wants to help or give back. Other groups may be formed by a health or religious organization, or even local or state governments. The key is knowing how to find the breast cancer support group or network that will best fit your needs. Some of the most common national breast cancer organizations/networks can provide information on support groups or resources. This appendix lists some supportive information, services organizations, and resources.

REMEMBER

This is a partial list of supportive resources available to breast cancer survivors. Please contact your local cancer society or cancer organizations for information on breast cancer supportive resources specific to your location.

American Breast Cancer Foundation (ABCF)

Find this organization at www.abcf.org and at 410-730-5105. On Facebook, check out www.facebook.com/americanbreastcancerfoundation, on Twitter it's at @TweetABCF, and on Instagram look for @americanbreastcancerfoundation. ABCF is a 501(c)(3) nonprofit organization.

The mission of the American Breast Cancer Foundation (ABCF) is to provide educational resources, access, and financial assistance to aid in the early detection, treatment, and survival of breast cancer for underserved and uninsured individuals, regardless of age or gender. This is achieved, in part, by the Breast Cancer Assistance Program (BCAP), the Community Partnership Program, and the newly designed Community Advocacy Program. For additional information, visit www. abcf.org.

The BCAP program and the Community Partnership Program help link patients with facilities and assistance in their own areas. The Community Advocacy Program is rooted in significant personal relationships with individuals, to assist them in gaining access to needed resources, services, and support.

The strategic platform provided by these programs serves as a link and referral system to local resources and information that is ethnically and linguistically appropriate to the needs of the individual. It is the goal of each of these programs to reduce disparities in access to diagnosis and the treatment of breast cancer. These interventions may lead to modification of negative factors and improve the survival rate of clients served.

American Cancer Society (ACS)

The society's online resources can be visited at www.cancer.org and at 1-800-227-2345. It offers the following information, services, and support programs for cancer patients and survivors:

>> Understanding your diagnosis

>> Finding and paying for treatment

>> Choosing and understanding treatments and their side effects

>> Taking part in clinical trials

>> Knowing what to do during and after treatment

>> Caring for children with cancer

For caregivers and family:

>> Understanding recurrence

>> Nearing end of life

>> Supporting people in your area

>> Using tools to help navigate treatment:

- Choosing your treatment team
- Being knowledgeable about insurance resources
- Reviewing survivorship care plans

American Society of Clinical Oncology (ASCO)

The society has a website at www.cancer.net or you can call 571-483-1780 or 1-888-651-3038. It offers a blog and information on services and treatments to make informed health decisions, including the following:

>> Knowing the different types of cancer

>> Navigating cancer care

>> Coping with cancer

>> Navigating survivorship

>> Doing research and advocacy

CancerCare

Check out www.cancercare.org or call 800-813-HOPE (4673). This organization provides emotional and practical support for individuals with cancer, caregivers, loved ones, and bereaved through the following means:

>> Counseling

>> Support groups

>> Educational workshops

>> Publications

>> Financial assistance

>> Community programs

4th Angel Patient and Caregiver Mentoring Program

You can visit this mentoring organization at www.4thangel.org. It provides free, one-on-one, confidential outreach and support from someone who has successfully made the same journey you are about to begin. The aim is to help in your journey toward recovery. You can participate in the following ways:

>> Requesting a mentor

>> Becoming a mentor

>> Monitoring caregivers

Livestrong.org

This organization at www.livestrong.org and 1-855-220-7777 provides information on direct services, community programs, and system change.

National Cancer Institute's Cancer Information Service

This information service is available at www.cancer.gov and at 1-800-4-CANCER (1-800-422-6237). It provides information on cancer questions within the following categories:

>> How to find cancer treatment centers

>> Cancer research and clinical trials

>> Cancer prevention

>> Risk factors

>> Early detection

>> Diagnosis and treatment

>> Living with cancer

>> Tissue donation

>> Quitting smoking

National Comprehensive Cancer Network (NCCN)

NCCN is accessible at www.nccn.org and at 215-690-0300. It provides patient and caregiver resources that are focused on advocacy and support groups, including in the following areas:

>> General cancer information/support

>> Blood and marrow transplants

>> Cancer and work

>> Fertility and pregnancy information

>> General prescription assistance

>> International/cultural support group

>> Test, imaging, and treatment-related patient information

>> Travel and lodging assistance

>> Age-related cancer support

>> Caregiving and survivorship

Susan G. Komen for the Cure

Online resource is at www.komen.org or by phone at 1-877-GO KOMEN (1-877-465-6636). The organization offers information, services, and support programs in the following areas:

>> Breast care helpline

>> Komen treatment assistance fund

- >> Interactive learning

- >> Komen educational materials and videos

- >> Questions to ask your doctor

- >> Screening reminder tool

- >> Komen message boards

- >> Breast cancer educational toolkits

- >> Funding for clinical trials/research

The ALERT

The ALERT (Australian Lymphoedema Education, Research, and Treatment) program at Macquarie University in Sydney, Australia, accessible at `https://www.mqhealth.org.au/hospital-clinics/lymphoedema-clinic`, consists of experienced multidisciplinary health professionals coming together to form a comprehensive clinical, research, and education service. The team aims to optimize positive outcomes for people at risk of or living with lymphoedema through excellence in assessment and management of the condition along the continuum. The ALERT program also offers conservative and surgical management of all types and stages of lymphoedema, supported by research and education initiatives, to provide the best care to patients.

Breast Cancer Network Australia

Breast Cancer Network Australia (BCNA), accessible at `www.bcna.org.au`, is Australia's peak national consumer organization for people affected by breast cancer. BCNA supports, informs, represents, and connects people whose lives have been affected by breast cancer.

BCNA's services include:

- >> Telephone helpline

- >> Range of high-quality print and digital resources, including the My Journey Kit for people with early breast cancer and Hope & Hurdles for people with metastatic breast cancer

- >> Online community

Cancer Australia

Cancer Australia, accessible at www.canceraustralia.gov.au, is the Australian government's national cancer agency, which aims to reduce the impact of cancer by providing leadership in cancer control, driving best practice care, funding priority research, strengthening data capacity, and promoting evidence-based cancer awareness and information.

Cancer Australia's website provides up-to-date, evidence-based information on breast cancer across the following areas:

>> Statistics

>> Types

>> Symptoms

>> Risk factors

>> Diagnosis

>> Treatment

>> Finding support

>> Living with breast cancer

>> Life after breast cancer

>> Breast cancer in men

>> Breast cancer in young women

MacMillan Cancer Support (U.K.)

This U.K resource is available at www.macmillan.org.uk and 0808 808 00 00. It provides information and support in the United Kingdom through education on the following topics:

>> Understanding what cancer is

>> Diagnosing symptoms, causes, and risk factors

>> Organizing the practical, work, and financial side

>> Treating cancer and knowing what to expect

>> Coping with and after cancer treatment

>> Offering resources and publications to order, download, or print

Canadian Cancer Society

Check out this society at http://support.cbcf.org and 1-888-778-3100. It provides support and information for Canadians in the following areas:

>> Breast health and cancer risk

>> Understanding breast cancer and diagnosis

>> Helping the newly diagnosed

>> Undergoing breast cancer treatment and knowing side effects

>> Navigating emotional and practical issues

>> Understanding breast reconstruction

>> Exploring hereditary breast and ovarian cancer (HBOC), metastatic breast cancer, and male breast cancer

>> Offering volunteer training programs for family and friends

>> Providing information about support groups

Cancer Chat Canada

This service is accessible at https://cancerchat.desouzainstitute.com and 1-844-725-2476. It offers online support groups in Canada.

RESOURCES FOR ETHNIC AND LINGUISTIC MINORITIES

- **Nueva Vida (www.nueva-vida.org):** Organization dedicated to informing, supporting, and empowering Latino families whose lives are affected by cancer

- **Sisters Network Inc. (www.sistersnetworkinc.org):** National African American breast cancer survivorship organization

- **Native American Cancer Network (natamcancer.org):** Improving the quality of cancer care and quality of life for all American Indian, Alaska Native, and First Nations cancer patients and their loved ones

- **Asian Pacific Islander National Cancer Survivors' Network (www.apiahf.org):** Network of cancer survivors, healthcare providers, and others concerned about cancer and survivorship in Asian American, Native Hawaiian, and Pacific Islander communities

Index

healthy lifestyle changes *(continued)*
  limiting or avoiding alcohol, 274–275
  losing weight, 267–268
  overcoming drug abuse, 276–277
  overview, 267
  quitting smoking, 272–274
  weight control, 280–283
Healthy People 2020, 257
heavy drinking
  pre-surgery concern, 118–119
  quitting before surgery, 121–122
  as risk factor, 21
hematologist, 122
hepatitis B virus (HBV), 165–166
HER2+, 74, 161, 193–194, 320
HER2/neu, 75, 320
HER2/neu receptors, 75, 106–107, 193–194
HER2/neu test, 74, 320
Herceptin, 106–107, 161–164, 194–195
heterocyclic amines (HCAs), 27
Hip-Hop Doc (Dr. Rani Whitfield), 274
Hispanic women, risk for breast cancer, 22
hormonal therapy. *See* endocrine therapy
hormone mimics, 31
hormone-receptor-negative, 75
hormone-receptor-positive, 75
hormone receptors, 190
hormone-replacement therapy (HRT), 30, 320
human papillomavirus (HPV), 165
humor, 304–305
hydrocodone, 125
hyperpigmentation, 232–233
hyperplasia, 71

I

ibuprofen, 122
idealized spiritual attribution, 214
imaging studies, 80
Imfinzi (durvalumab), 167
immediate breast reconstruction, 173–175
immune system, 275

immunizations, 199
immunoliposomes, 169
immunotherapy, 164
incidence rate, 20
indicators of breast cancer
  breast aches and pains, 40–41
  breast size and shape monitoring, 34–35
  decrease in breast size, 35
  increase in breast size, 35
  lumps and bumps, 39–40
  nipple changes, 40–43
  overview, 9–10, 33–34
  skin changes, 36–38
infections in breast, 38
infertility. *See also* fertility preservation
  BETTER model approach, 257–259
  breast cancer and, 250
  cancer treatment and, 212–213, 251–253
  causes of, 250–251
  complementary and alternative treatments, 256–257
  defined, 250, 320
  early menopause and, 254
  emotional side of, 258
  fear of, 212–213
  good clinical care practice for, 257
  permanent, 253
  social determinants of, 251
  temporary, 253
  tissue banking for fertility preservation, 254–256
inflammatory breast cancer, 12, 73, 320
infraclavicular nodes, 320
injection site, 232
inner peace, 225–226
in-situ, 71
Institute of Medicine, 258
Institutional Review Board (IRB), 110
insurance, 122
intensity modulated radiotherapy (IMRT), 129–130
internal mammary nodes, 320
intimacy, 262–263
intraductal breast papilloma, 320–321

intraductal carcinoma, 320
intraductal papilloma (IP), 42, 73, 320
intraoperative radiation, 130
intravenous infusion (IV), 123
invasive (or infiltrating cancer)
  age and death, 20
  defined, 14, 72, 321
invasive ductal carcinoma (IDC), 11, 73, 321
invasive lobular carcinoma (ILC), 321
in vitro fertilization, 255
iron deficiency, 41

J
jogging
  light, 271
  long-distance, 272
juice, 282

K
Kadcyla (T-DM1), 109, 161
Keytruda (pembrolizumab), 166
killer T-cells, 165, 321
Klinefelter syndrome, 21

L
laboratory tests, 80
lactose intolerance, 248
lapatinib, 109, 162
late menopause, 23
Latin word for crab, 13
latissimus dorsi flap, 181
laughter, benefits of, 304–305
learning to listen, 303
letrozole, 162
licorice, 200
life after breast cancer (ten ways)
  adopting attitude of gratitude, 308
  cancer survivorship plan, 314
  enjoying the moment, 308
  knowing you deserve to be happy, 308–309

learning about health, 309–310
  learning to be in the here and now, 311
  learning to pick battles, 310–311
  managing physical changes, 312–313
  positive self-talk and conversations, 311
  screening tests and schedules, 315–316
  self-acceptance, 313–314
liver
  cirrhosis of, 21
  effect of alcohol on, 274–275
Livestrong Cancer Policy Platform Federal Priority Report (2011), 258
Livestrong.org, 330
Living Beyond Breast Cancer, 259
lobes, 8
lobular carcinoma (cancer of lobules), 12
lobular carcinoma in situ (LCIS), 12–13, 71, 73, 321
lobular neoplasia, 321
lobules, 8, 10, 321
locally advanced cancer, 82
local recurrence, 82
losing weight. *See* weight control
lumpectomy, 66, 114
lupus, 82
lying in a meadow (visualization exercise), 222
lymph, 321
lymphatic system, 239
lymphatic vessels, 321
lymphedema
  causes of, 238
  defined, 115, 238
  fitness and exercise advice for, 241
  overview, 137
  preventative measures, 240–241
  resources for management of, 241
  symptoms of, 230
  treatment of, 239–240
Lymphedema Resources, Inc., 241
lymphedema therapist, 135
Lymphedivas, 241
lymph fluid, 115
lymph nodes, 9, 10, 321

P

prolactin, 7, 42, 323

prolactinoma, 42

Prolia (denosumab), 196–197

prophylactic mastectomy, 100, 114, 173, 323

propoxyphene, 125

prostate cancer screening (for men), 316

prosthesis, 182

protective factor, 323

protein-receptor, 323

Provenge, 166

psychiatrist, 125

psychosocial concerns
anxiety, 210
concern for children, 208
depression, 209
fear of cancer recurrence, 209
overview, 207–208
physical impact of cancer and, 208
spirituality, 214
support groups, 215–216
work and home life concerns, 210–214

Q

quick meals, 282–283

Quitter (app), 274

R

race, as risk factor, 21–22

radial scar, 73

radiation
cough, 138
defined, 323
exposure, 21, 30–31

radiation oncologist, 16, 104, 125, 128, 131

radiation physicist, 131

radiation technologist, 58, 104–105

radiation therapy
adjuvant or additional, 128
for advanced breast cancer, 201–202
bone weakening after, 139
boost, 130

brachytherapy, 130
change in breast size/consistency after, 134, 137–138
contouring in, 131
defined, 102–103
dry cough, 138
exercises after, 135–137
fibrosis over the ribs during, 138
fibrosis under the arm after, 138
fractions, 129
hair loss and, 230–232
hair loss in armpit or chest area after, 138
heart problems after, 139
how it works, 128–129
as injection, 201
intensity modulated, 129–130
intraoperative, 130
lymphedema after, 137
NCCN guidelines, 128
neoadjuvant, 128
overview, 17, 127–128
pain in breast area after, 135
planning for, 131–132
post-radiation skincare, 133–134
questions to ask before, 132
respiratory gating, 130
side effects of, 103–104, 134–135, 137–139, 201–202
skincare during, 104–105
skin discoloration after, 232
skin reactions to, 134
swelling/edema of breast after, 135
tenderness over the rib during, 138
things to do before, 132–133
tingling, numbness, and pain in the arm after, 139
tiredness and fatigue after, 137
types of, 129–130

radical mastectomy, 323

radiologist, 16, 58, 76, 323

radon, 31

randomization, 110

transducer, 59

transitional survivorship, 288

transverse rectus abdominis myocutaneous (TRAM) flap, 179–180

trastuzumab
  for advanced breast cancer, 194–195
  HER2/neu protein inhibition by, 74, 161
  precision medicine and, 106–107
  side effects, 163–164

trauma recall, 214

treatment
  of advanced breast cancer, 18
  breast reconstruction, 101–102
  breast surgery, 16
  chemotherapy, 17, 105–106
  clinical trials, 109–111
  doctor's recommendation, 96
  endocrine therapy, 17, 106
  factors in selection of, 95
  hormonal therapy, 106
  infertility and, 251–253
  options, 15–16
  overview, 93–96
  physical changes after, 312–313
  planning, 15–18
  prognosis, 94
  radiation, 17
  radiation therapy, 102–105
  surgeries, 96–100
  survival rate, 93–94
  targeted therapy, 106–109
  types of, 95

triclosan, 31

triple negative breast cancers, 21–22, 75, 326

tumor
  benign, 10, 64, 71
  defined, 326
  grade of, 15, 81
  local, 81
  malignant, 10, 72
  poorly differentiated, 81

  regional, 81
  well-differentiated, 81

turmeric, 201

Tykerb (lapatinib), 162

Tylenol (acetaminophen/paracetamol), 122

Tylenol #3 (codeine), 125

tyrosine kinase inhibitors, 162

U

ultrasound, 59–61, 326

ultrasound-guided core biopsy, 66

underarm
  lymph nodes in, 9
  shaving before surgery, 121

underweight, 28

undifferentiated tumor, 81

universal connectedness, 214

urinary catheter, 123

usual ductal hyperplasia (UDH), 71

V

varenicline, 273

verapamil, 42

vesicants, 232

Vicodin (hydrocodone), 125

vinca alkaloids, 144, 145

visualization exercise, 222

vitamin A, 200

vitamin C, 200

vitamin E, 200

voicemail, 305

W

walking, 230

wall climbing, 136

weight control
  activities for, 280
  being realistic, 268
  changing mind, 268

About the Authors

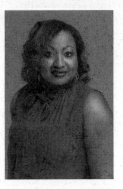

Marshalee George, PhD, MSPH, MSN, AOCNP®, CRNP, is faculty research associate and oncology nurse practitioner at Johns Hopkins University School of Medicine and adjunct DNP nursing faculty at Johns Hopkins University School of Nursing, Baltimore, Maryland. She obtained her bachelor of nursing degree at Coppin State University and went on to complete her master's in nursing with specialization as a nurse practitioner and clinical nurse specialist in oncology and adult primary care at the University of Pennsylvania in Philadelphia. She has a passion for community medicine and engaging diverse populations to improve population health and reduce health disparities. She went on to complete a master's in public health with concentration in community health and subsequent doctorate in public health with specialization in program planning, education, and development at Walden University, Minnesota. She completed a three-year traineeship at Johns Hopkins University Bloomberg School of Public Health, focused on reducing health and cancer disparities in underserved and vulnerable populations.

Dr. George is board certified in oncology and primary care. She has 20 years' experience in oncology (medical and surgical), research/clinical trials, and care coordination. She has experience in grant writing, program development, outcome measures, and community engagement, education, and advocacy. She has clinically managed breast cancer patients at Johns Hopkins Breast Centers in Baltimore for the past ten years. She is the founder of the first Johns Hopkins Bayview Medical Center Breast Cancer Survivor's Community Program. Since 2014, this program has been providing survivorship care planning and implementation, including patient educational and self-management support for survivors to learn how to improve cancer outcomes and well-being post breast cancer. She also holds adjunct faculty positions at Southern California University and the University of the Southern Caribbean in Trinidad & Tobago, West Indies.

Dr. George has held several leadership positions as clinical director in primary care practices and she is a medical entrepreneur. She also embraces volunteerism by serving as a board member of Caribbean Medical Providers Practicing Abroad (CMPPA), a 501(c)(3) volunteer organization focused on improving medical care in the Caribbean and Caribbean immigrant populations in the United States.

Dr. George is known as a community-minded practitioner. She excels in patient care especially focusing on health promotion, illness prevention, chronic disease management (diabetes, hypertension, stroke, and more), and cancer awareness and survivorship. She also coaches individuals and entities through screening, diagnosis, treatment, and survivorship processes from various healthcare systems locally, nationally, and internationally. She has published in the areas of breast cancer disparities and survivorship care. She serves as a reviewer for *Clinical Journal of Oncology Nursing* and the Oncology Nursing Society. She is a member of the American Academy of Nurse Practitioners, Oncology Nursing Society, and American Psychosocial Oncology Society.

Dr. George is married and a mother of two children: Annalyse, a science, math, and dance enthusiast in the 12th grade; and Alessio, an avid preschooler fan of Hot Wheels and animated characters. She lives in the beautiful state of Maryland, where Francis Scott Key wrote the U.S. national anthem, "The Star-Spangled Banner," in 1814.

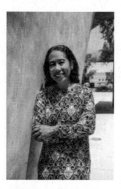

Kimlin Tam Ashing, PhD, is professor and founding director of the Center of Community Alliance for Research and Education (CCARE) at City of Hope Medical Center. She received her doctorate in clinical psychology from the University of Colorado, Boulder. As an advocate-scientist, her work is advancing population health. She is a population behavioral scientist working to develop and implement evidenced-based, culturally, clinically, and community-responsive health improvement interventions. Her mission is to engage advocates and civil society in science to speed up and ensure the public benefit of biomedical research and advancements.

Dr. Ashing holds several national leadership roles within the African-Caribbean Cancer Consortium; National Advisory Council for the Asian Pacific Islander Native Hawaiian Cancer Survivors Network, and the Young Survival Coalition; and the Executive Council of American Cancer Society, Los Angeles. She is a life member of the Association of Black Psychologists and a licensed clinical psychologist. She served as board member and continues on the Scientific Committee of the American Psychosocial Oncology Society. She serves as scientific advisor to Latinas Contra Cancer, Caribbean Medical Providers Practicing Abroad, and Army of Women. She is a scientific partner with the Association of Black Women Physicians, Los Angeles chapter, and the Take Action of Health Initiative, a community benefits partnership among National Urban League, Anthem, and Pfizer. She was awarded the prestigious Fox Award for advancing the field of psychooncology by the International Psychooncology Society and is a member of the Human Rights Taskforce. She sits on the Minority in Cancer Research Council of the American Association of Cancer Researchers — the largest body of cancer researchers in the world.

Dr. Ashing is a notable leader in examining health disparities, cancer inequities, survivorship, and quality of life. She has published over 80 articles and book chapters. Her scholarship is to understand how cultural, ethnic, socio-ecological, structural, and systemic contexts influence health- and patient-centered outcomes, including mortality, morbidity, distress, symptoms, and quality of life. She applies this knowledge to implement interventions to improve well-being and reduce health inequities.

Dedication

We dedicate this book to all our patients and study participants who have taught us and showed us the full experience of survivorship. This book is our gift, as healthcare professionals and daughters, to all personally touched by cancer.

Author's Acknowledgments

I would like to thank God for blessing me with wisdom, knowledge, and understanding to provide the care and education that I enjoy giving to cancer survivors. I thank my husband, Barry, my children, Annalyse and Alessio, and my mother, Ina, and three siblings, Victor, Staceyann, and Lisa, for their dedication and support and for taking on so many more of my responsibilities while writing this book. To Dr. Kimlin Tam Ashing, your mentorship, friendship, and support have been a stronghold in my professional growth in the field of psychooncology and my ability to better assess and address cancer survivors' distress in clinical settings.

To my colleagues at Johns Hopkins Sidney Kimmel Comprehensive Cancer Center — Johns Hopkins Breast Center, I thank you for your support in providing peer review of this book to ensure that the readers have the most up-to-date, relevant, and evidence-based information for treating breast cancer and living well beyond treatment. I would also like to thank my Caribbean Medical Providers Practicing Abroad (CMPPA) network for helping me to understand the global impact that education and medical volunteerism can have on improving the lives and health outcomes of cancer survivors where medical resources are limited.

— Dr. Marshalee George

I thank God from whom all blessings flow. I have been transformed through the cancer journey, as my mother and father were both diagnosed with cancers and their lives were cut short by this disease. To honor my mother and father, I have dedicated my life's work to understanding the needs of cancer survivors and studying how to enhance quality of care, quality of life, and well-being among those affected by cancer.

I am grateful to my family — my seven siblings and my three children, Josh, Ajorin, and Kemi — whose love and constant support give meaning and belonging.

I thank my colleagues at City of Hope Medical Center for their professional review. I thank Dr. Marshalee George, who epitomizes professionalism and generosity. My respect for her and our friendship deepened in the process of writing together.

— Dr. Kimlin Tam Ashing

Special thanks to Katherine Mele of ABCF for all her help during this project. And special thanks to our sci-med peer reviewers:

Vered Stearns, MD, professor of oncology, co-director, Breast and Ovarian Cancer Program, breast cancer research chair in oncology, the Sidney Kimmel Comprehensive Cancer Center at Johns Hopkins, associate medical director, Johns Hopkins Singapore

Veronica C. Jones, MD, breast surgeon, assistant clinical professor, Division of Surgical Oncology, Department of Surgery, City of Hope Comprehensive Cancer Center

Lisa K. Jacobs, MD, MSPH, FACS, associate professor of surgery, associate professor of oncology, Surgical Oncology Division, Johns Hopkins Breast Center, Johns Hopkins University School of Medicine

Cristiane Decat Bergerot, PhD, clinical psychologist, Department of Medical Oncology & Experimental Therapeutics, City of Hope Comprehensive Cancer Center

David Eisner, MD, assistant professor of radiology, Division of Breast Imaging, Johns Hopkins University School of Medicine

Publisher's Acknowledgments

Acquisitions Editor: Tracy Boggier
Editor: Corbin Collins
Technical Editor: Mackenzie Goodwin, MD

Production Editor: Selvakumaran Rajendiran
Cover Photos: © photo story/Shutterstock

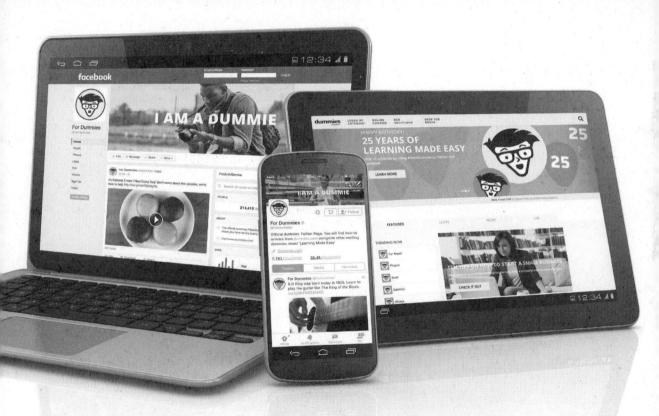

Take dummies with you everywhere you go!

Whether you are excited about e-books, want more from the web, must have your mobile apps, or are swept up in social media, dummies makes everything easier.

Find us online!

dummies.com

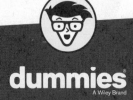

Leverage the power

Dummies is the global leader in the reference category and one of the most trusted and highly regarded brands in the world. No longer just focused on books, customers now have access to the dummies content they need in the format they want. Together we'll craft a solution that engages your customers, stands out from the competition, and helps you meet your goals.

Advertising & Sponsorships

Connect with an engaged audience on a powerful multimedia site, and position your message alongside expert how-to content. Dummies.com is a one-stop shop for free, online information and know-how curated by a team of experts.

- Targeted ads
- Video
- Email Marketing
- Microsites
- Sweepstakes sponsorship

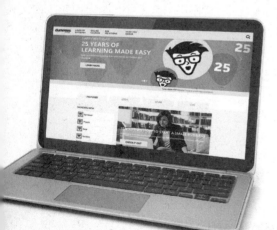

20 MILLION PAGE VIEWS EVERY SINGLE MONTH

15 MILLION UNIQUE VISITORS PER MONTH

43% OF ALL VISITORS ACCESS THE SITE VIA THEIR MOBILE DEVICES

700,000 NEWSLETTER SUBSCRIPTIONS TO THE INBOXES OF *300,000* UNIQUE INDIVIDUALS EVERY WEEK

# of dummies

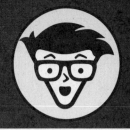

Custom Publishing

Reach a global audience in any language by creating a solution that will differentiate you from competitors, amplify your message, and encourage customers to make a buying decision.

- Apps
- Books
- eBooks
- Video
- Audio
- Webinars

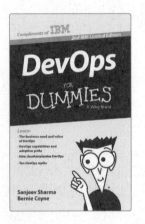
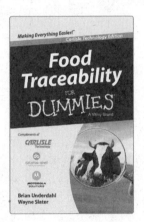
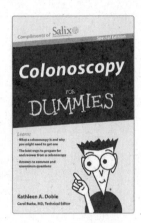
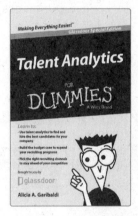

Brand Licensing & Content

Leverage the strength of the world's most popular reference brand to reach new audiences and channels of distribution.

For more information, visit dummies.com/biz

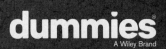

PERSONAL ENRICHMENT

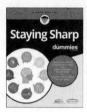 **Staying Sharp** dummies
9781119187790
USA $26.00
CAN $31.99
UK £19.99

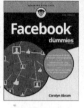 **Facebook** dummies
Carolyn Abram
9781119179030
USA $21.99
CAN $25.99
UK £16.99

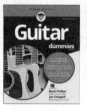 **Guitar** dummies
Mark Phillips
Jon Chappell
9781119293354
USA $24.99
CAN $29.99
UK £17.99

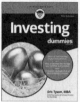 **Investing** dummies
Eric Tyson, MBA
9781119293347
USA $22.99
CAN $27.99
UK £16.99

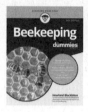 **Beekeeping** dummies
Howland Blackiston
9781119310068
USA $22.99
CAN $27.99
UK £16.99

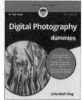 **Digital Photography** dummies
Julie Adair King
9781119235606
USA $24.99
CAN $29.99
UK £17.99

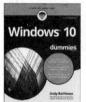 **Meditation** dummies
Stephan Bodian
9781119251163
USA $24.99
CAN $29.99
UK £17.99

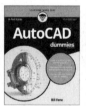 **Pregnancy** ALL-IN-ONE dummies
6 Books
9781119235491
USA $26.99
CAN $31.99
UK £19.99

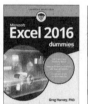 **Samsung Galaxy S7** dummies
Bill Hughes
9781119279952
USA $24.99
CAN $29.99
UK £17.99

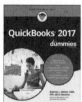 **iPhone** dummies
Edward C. Baig
Bob "Dr. Mac" LeVitus
9781119283133
USA $24.99
CAN $29.99
UK £17.99

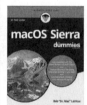 **Crocheting** dummies
Karen Manthey
Susan Brittain
9781119287117
USA $24.99
CAN $29.99
UK £16.99

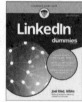 **Nutrition** dummies
Carol Ann Rinzler
9781119130246
USA $22.99
CAN $27.99
UK £16.99

PROFESSIONAL DEVELOPMENT

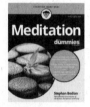 **Windows 10** dummies
Andy Rathbone
9781119311041
USA $24.99
CAN $29.99
UK £17.99

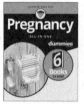 **AutoCAD** dummies
Bill Fane
9781119255796
USA $39.99
CAN $47.99
UK £27.99

 Excel 2016 dummies
Greg Harvey, PhD
9781119293439
USA $26.99
CAN $31.99
UK £19.99

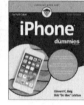 **QuickBooks 2017** dummies
Stephen L. Nelson, MBA, CPA, MS in Taxation
9781119281467
USA $26.99
CAN $31.99
UK £19.99

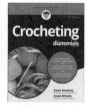 **macOS Sierra** dummies
Bob "Dr. Mac" LeVitus
9781119280651
USA $29.99
CAN $35.99
UK £21.99

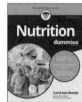 **LinkedIn** dummies
Joel Elad, MBAs
9781119251132
USA $24.99
CAN $29.99
UK £17.99

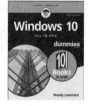 **Windows 10** ALL-IN-ONE dummies
10 Books in one!
Woody Leonhard
9781119310563
USA $34.00
CAN $41.99
UK £24.99

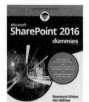 **SharePoint 2016** dummies
Rosemarie Withee
Ken Withee
9781119181705
USA $29.99
CAN $35.99
UK £21.99

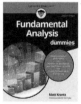 **Fundamental Analysis** dummies
Matt Krantz
9781119263593
USA $26.99
CAN $31.99
UK £19.99

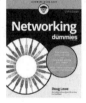 **Networking** dummies
Doug Lowe
9781119257769
USA $29.99
CAN $35.99
UK £21.99

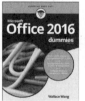 **Office 2016** dummies
Wallace Wang
9781119293477
USA $26.99
CAN $31.99
UK £19.99

 Office 365 dummies
Rosemarie Withee
Ken Withee
Jennifer Reed
9781119265313
USA $24.99
CAN $29.99
UK £17.99

 Salesforce.com dummies
Liz Kao
Jon Paz
9781119239314
USA $29.99
CAN $35.99
UK £21.99

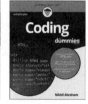 **Coding** dummies
Nikhil Abraham
9781119293323
USA $29.99
CAN $35.99
UK £21.99

dummies.com

dummies A Wiley Brand

Learning Made Easy

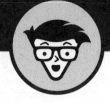

ACADEMIC

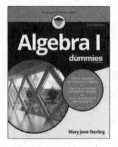

9781119293576
USA $19.99
CAN $23.99
UK £15.99

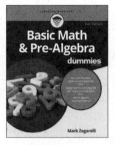

9781119293637
USA $19.99
CAN $23.99
UK £15.99

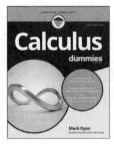

9781119293491
USA $19.99
CAN $23.99
UK £15.99

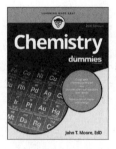

9781119293460
USA $19.99
CAN $23.99
UK £15.99

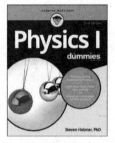

9781119293590
USA $19.99
CAN $23.99
UK £15.99

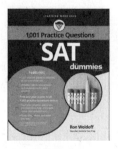

9781119215844
USA $26.99
CAN $31.99
UK £19.99

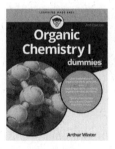

9781119293378
USA $22.99
CAN $27.99
UK £16.99

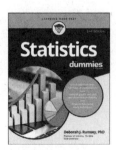

9781119293521
USA $19.99
CAN $23.99
UK £15.99

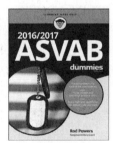

9781119239178
USA $18.99
CAN $22.99
UK £14.99

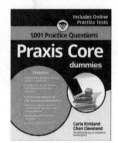

9781119263883
USA $26.99
CAN $31.99
UK £19.99

Available Everywhere Books Are Sold

dummies.com

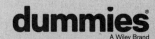

Small books for big imaginations

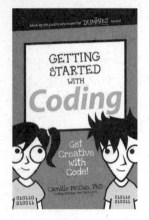

GETTING STARTED WITH **Coding**
Get Creative with Code!
Camille McCue, PhD

9781119177173
USA $9.99
CAN $9.99
UK £8.99

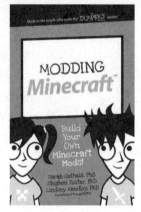

MODDING **Minecraft™**
Build Your Own Minecraft Mods!
Sarah Guthals, PhD
Stephen Foster, PhD
Lindsey Handley, PhD

9781119177272
USA $9.99
CAN $9.99
UK £8.99

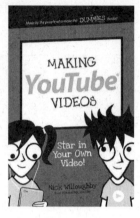

MAKING **YouTube** VIDEOS
Star in Your Own Video!
Nick Willoughby

9781119177241
USA $9.99
CAN $9.99
UK £8.99

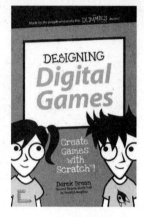

DESIGNING **Digital Games**
Create Games with Scratch™!
Derek Breen

9781119177210
USA $9.99
CAN $9.99
UK £8.99

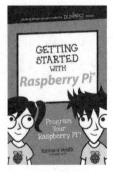

GETTING STARTED WITH **Raspberry Pi™**
Program Your Raspberry Pi!
Richard Wentk

9781119262657
USA $9.99
CAN $9.99
UK £6.99

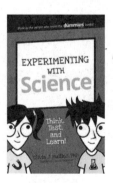

EXPERIMENTING WITH **Science**
Think, Test, and Learn!
Silvia J. Palillos, PhD

9781119291336
USA $9.99
CAN $9.99
UK £6.99

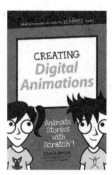

CREATING **Digital Animations**
Animate Stories with Scratch™!
Derek Breen

9781119233527
USA $9.99
CAN $9.99
UK £6.99

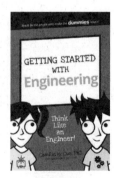

GETTING STARTED WITH **Engineering**
Think Like an Engineer!
Camille McCue, PhD

9781119291220
USA $9.99
CAN $9.99
UK £6.99

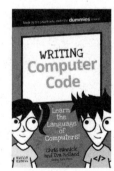

WRITING **Computer Code**
Learn the Language of Computers!
Chris Minnick and Eva Holland

9781119177302
USA $9.99
CAN $9.99
UK £8.99

Unleash Their Creativity

dummies.com

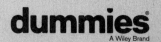

A Wiley Brand